Praise for *Seahorses*

"By looking with love through a gender-expansive lens, *Seahorses* shifts the narrative of reproductive health and justice for all of us. The stories uplift and dive into the honest and nuanced spectrum of human emotion: tenderly understanding grief, joy, rage, growth, intimacy. As we are situated in a violent and precarious political landscape with regard to body autonomy and gender, this book is needed now more than ever."
—Syan Rose, creator of *Our Work Is Everywhere: An Illustrated Oral History of Queer and Trans Resistance*

"*Seahorses* illustrates how choosing to be pregnant (or not) as a transgender person can be a bold and revolutionary act. With far-right forces chipping away at our reproductive and gender-affirming rights, this book is a must-read. It powerfully demonstrates that body autonomy, including the right to pregnancy and reproductive justice, is at the heart of true gender-affirming justice."
—Zane McNeill, editor of *Y'all Means All: The Emerging Voices Queering Appalachia* and coeditor of *Be Gay, Do Crime: Everyday Acts of Queer Resistance and Rebellion*

"*Seahorses* is a groundbreaking treasure! The first of its kind to compile the invaluable breadth of knowledge and wisdom held beyond the narrow confines of mainstream pregnancy and gender, making it not only an essential, diverse resource but also a thought-provoking, heart-expanding chronicle, voicing overlooked and underrepresented experiences. Everyone should read this book, regardless of gender or sexual orientation."
—Miles Borrero, author of *Beautiful Monster: A Becoming*

"Open this book, take the invitation to discover the power of community and family, because finally we have a parenting book for all families; in fact, everyone should read this book."
—Tomas Moniz, editor of *Rad Dad* and *Rad Families* and author of *All Friends Are Necessary*

"This book is a gift to the world."
—Freddy McConnell, author of *Little Seahorse and the Big Question*

"In a world often defined by rigid boundaries and societal expectations, this book emerges as a vibrant celebration of our diverse identities and the multifaceted experiences of trans, nonbinary, and gender-expansive individuals. More than a collection of stories, it is a testament to resilience, community, and the transformative power of love.

"Through heartfelt narratives and poignant reflections, readers are invited into the intimate journeys of those who navigate pregnancy and parenthood against the backdrop of a rapidly changing world. With each page, the voices within affirm our existence and the profound beauty of our unique paths.

"This book is a beacon of hope, a declaration that there is space for everyone. It stands as an artifact of our times, capturing the struggles, the triumphs, and the relentless pursuit of joy amidst adversity. May it inspire you to embrace your story, find solace in shared experiences, and kindle the spark of belonging in every heart."
—Trystan Reese, author of *How We Do Family: From Adoption to Trans Pregnancy, What We Learned About Love and LGBTQ Parenthood*

Seahorses

Trans, Nonbinary, and Gender-Expansive Pregnancy

Edited by Simon Knaphus

Foreword by Jacoby Ballard

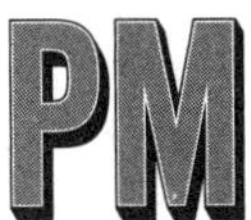

Seahorses: Trans, Nonbinary, and Gender-Expansive Pregnancy

ISBN: 979-8-88744-128-3 (paperback)
ISBN: 979-8-88744-129-0 (ebook)
LCCN: 2025931280

Cover by John Yates / stealworks.com
Cover art by Sam Vanbelle
Interior design by briandesign

10 9 8 7 6 5 4 3 2 1

PM Press
PO Box 23912
Oakland, CA 94623
www.pmpress.org

Printed in the USA.

I believe that telling our stories, first to ourselves and then to one another and the world, is a revolutionary act.

—Janet Mock, *Redefining Realness: My Path to Womanhood, Identity, Love & So Much More*

Contents

A Note to Readers

This book was written by and for trans, nonbinary, and gender-expansive people who have experienced or will experience pregnancy. If this is you, welcome in—please make yourself at home.

If this is not you, you are welcome as a guest. Thank you for sharing your time with us! Our journeys would not be complete without the open-hearted support of our loved ones, and our allies are essential. If you find yourself struggling to approach our stories with tenderness, please set this book down and come join us again when you are ready.

A note on style and spelling: This book retains the preference of the individual contributors when it comes to variations of identity terms, such as *nonbinary* and *non-binary*.

Foreword

Jacoby Ballard

What you hold in your hands is sacred. These stories have been told in small circles at transgender health conferences, in doctors' and midwives' offices, and among friends, but this is a new public offering of our trans and nonbinary journey with fertility, conception, pregnancy, and parenthood. Trans folks have existed throughout time and across cultures, and so I must believe that we have had families and borne children throughout time and across cultures. Being transparents is not new, but here you have a public offering of our sweat, tears, laughter, and orgasms. That is new.

Part of queer culture is to challenge conventional notions: about who to love, what makes a family, what words work for one's body or parental titles, what it is to be trans or not, what makes a "man" or a "woman," which then we can apply to fertility and conception processes, fetal loss, birth work culture, what is considered "natural" or hardcore, or not, and the possibilities and challenges of parenting. This superpower that we possess is now an offering to the world. We are creating the world that we want to live in, a world that makes more room for trans and nonbinary authenticity, and therefore that of everyone, a world where we are not expected to compromise any part of who we are. We present our authenticity by simply existing, and in this anthology, we tell our truths through the family-making process. Both gender transition and pregnancy are spiritual experiences as well as "physical transformations which offer opportunities for autonomy and surrender," author Halo Dawn declares.

The authors of this anthology bravely discuss pregnancy journeys that must go through obstacle courses of transphobia and misogyny, which are being politically stoked by the *Dobbs* decision to repeal *Roe v. Wade* and abortion access as well as well as encountering an annual record-breaking quantity of anti-trans bills in state legislatures. We are living the question: What is the impact on quality health care for trans birthing people if our lives and health care choices are being condemned and eliminated through policy decisions and the implementation of those policies?

Some authors herein are solo parents, some are partnered, some became partnered through pregnancy and parenting, and others experienced divorce as they maneuvered the parenting path. Some authors write about their experience of miscarriage or abortion, the former a loss made more sorrowful by a lack of choice and the latter a choice to release life when the timing isn't ripe to be a good parent. Some people had home births, and some had a medically directed experience from the beginning. Just like being queer or being trans, birth experience is a universe and we are all stars!

A gift that we offer our children is our intention and purpose in bringing them into the world. There is significant forethought in bringing our children earthside, in how we find the necessary components of egg, sperm, and uterus. As you will read, we deeply contemplate our parenting choices and life choices, considering what we are teaching our children about the gender binary, race and racism, ableism and disability. As we interact with the reproductive industry and birth work world, as well as the world of parenting, we confront arenas laden with misogyny, transphobia, heterosexism, racism, and ableism, which we may have largely avoided before trying to conceive, being pregnant, and parenting. We face microaggressions about who the parent/gestator is as we seek trans-affirming care, and we also encounter anticipated complications of the medical-industrial complex that any ciswoman might face regarding being believed and trusted about what she says about her body (or not, as is so often the case). As trans people, our realness and validity are often challenged, and our experience in the reproductive health industry splices that doubt with medical misogyny and transphobia.

As trans birthing people, chestfeeders, and parents, we inherited the feminism of midwives, doulas, and birth centers who have done potent political work to center the birthing body and one's self-determination. Simon Knaphus expresses, "Pregnancy and its institutions (midwifery, prenatal yoga, online spaces, birth classes) are places where women's knowledge and power have more room to breathe inside patriarchy, thanks to decades of feminist activist work." In these stories of those living and birthing outside the gender binary, you will read about our gratitude for this feminist reproductive justice history as well as our exclusion, disappointment, and grief. In some of our stories, we have been received with willingness and interest but a lack of experience with trans people (so we had to be the educators), and in a few of these spaces the others involved have done the work to welcome and anticipate us. An author wrote about their doula even rerecording pregnancy meditations that she gives out to clients to be gender-inclusive for a trans client. Many birthing centers and maternity wards have also been painful sites of misgendering or the denial of care for trans people.

This anthology contains a feeling of connection to other birthing parents and babywearers across a myriad of genders, time, and distance. I still feel a sense of fellowship with every other parent that I encounter, no matter the different children that we are raising or our different parenting choices. Birth is a human experience and serves to humanize trans people in a unique way. Everyone was born to someone who gave birth in some way.

What We Navigate in Trans Pregnancy

As trans and nonbinary birthing parents, we give birth into relationships that have withstood not only all normal relationship challenges but also homophobia and transphobia, as well as varied paths of transition. The authors here navigate the question of starting testosterone or getting pregnant, along with the complexity of having to come off testosterone and have a different hormonal arrangement in the body. They discuss the choice of breast/chestfeeding, with some of us having the mammary tissue to feed a child and some of us having had top surgery that removed that tissue and thereby removed that option. Some of us even had chest surgery at a time when some mammary tissue was left in the chest to mimic the shape of a cisgender male's chest, and that tissue can engorge at birth but not release breast milk because the ducts were severed in surgery.

The authors discuss how pregnancy impacts how one feels in one's trans identity, in some cases bringing that identity into question, and in some cases deeply affirming it in a way that nothing else had. Some authors reveal their dissociation or dysphoria when they were pregnant, while others felt deeply themselves. Many of the authors express an awe at being able to create life, a love of the opportunity of this body that was granted a uterus and ovaries. Other authors reflect on the experience of being cis-assumed, their transness invisiblized as their pregnancy became more visible. "We face a season of invisibility and erasure while simultaneously working to grow life (and sometimes while also coping with unspeakable loss)," says Aakash Kishore. Some people who regularly, pre-pregnancy, experienced gender dysphoria as a part of life offer up pregnancy as a lived experience in which the body could not be ignored. Authors here had a fear and experience of being misgendered during birth, and some authors tell incredibly trans-affirming birth stories. And some stories reflect an impatience with transphobia through and because of their pregnancy, leading them to speak up and intervene more often.

As a prenatal yoga teacher, I hear many of my trans students talk about how being recognizably pregnant can compromise our safety and create openings for misgendering, while when being invisibly pregnant, passing as a man, one's pregnancy is overlooked. Each of us have to choose how to navigate that. I was on a New York subway when five months pregnant and contemplated for the entire ride either outing myself by asking for a seat or withstanding the toss and turn and risking a fall if I remained standing.

As we bring children into the world, we may face exclusion in a community where so many of us have found solace. The authors here reveal both the support and care of the queer community as well as, sometimes, the judgment and exclusion, being dismissed as "breeders" and "normies" for having children. Some authors experienced more surprise from the queer community in revealing that they were pregnant than they had in revealing their transition path. This invites self-reflection for our entire community: Who is welcome, and who is not? What is included in queerness, and what is outside the umbrella?

Also present in this anthology is the complex relationship that many of us have with our own parents, some of whom have embraced us as trans people and some of whom have shown waves or consistent rejection of our declaration of who we are. This means that some grandparents are a welcome part of pregnancy and birth, some want to be included in their grandchild's birth while keeping their transphobia intact and so are not invited to the party, and some extricate themselves during or preceding birth because of their maintenance of the gender binary, homophobia, and transphobia. Each of us navigate this in different ways and with varied tool sets, some of us with clear boundaries and some of us giving opportunities for our parents to demonstrate their own growth so that they are welcome as active participants in our children's lives.

The authors discuss the insight that one's trans identity brings to parenthood. Many authors here are raising "theybies," exploring gender-expansive parenting that allows our children any choice of toy, clothing, hobby, embodiment, or interest. We discuss how easily our children embrace our genders, not inculcated by the gender binary and cisnormative world, seeing us as "normal" or "natural" from the beginning. We may use different parenting labels, from "baba" to "appa," "maddie" to "dama," that don't strictly adhere to the gender binary, and our children may have to do some translation for friends not raised in a queer family.

The discussion sessions, where authors conversed with one another on various topics, are particularly rich, offering reflections on fashion, thoughts about words they used for their processes, and advice and recommendations for fellow trans and nonbinary parents. The authors explore questions together about embodiment, spirituality, reproductive choice, whether providers were previously trans-informed or not, and more.

We want to report—and welcome you into—a growth of queer- and trans-affirming birth spaces in the past twenty years, including the Pregnant Together community, the book *Babymaking for Everybody*, the Queer and Transgender Midwives Association, the *Masculine Birth Ritual* podcast, and the Queer Doula Network, as well as the more binary but queer-oriented resources that preceded these. Birth work is expanding, responding to and because of our own stories and advocacy and the organizing of the reproductive justice movement led by women of color. As my colleague angel Kyodo williams instructed me years ago, "If there's something you want and don't see in a space, that is because it's your offering to make." Trans and nonbinary birthers and parents, along with our providers and communities, are doing just that, and we leave behind a legacy and birth work world more open and inclusive than it ever has been before, through and despite our own challenges, and certainly due to our queer creativity in family making.

Introduction

This book feels like a celebration to me, a declaration of our existence, a welcoming and an artifact from our community—our communities. It is a gathering in of readers, writers, and families. I am positively thrilled to have worked with the fine people whose stories speak from these pages! I hope that you will read these stories and know that whoever you are, there is room for you.

I started trying to write and gather contributions for this book twelve years ago, when my kids were seven and two. It is the book I wanted to find when I started trying to get pregnant. I wasn't able to bring it to fruition through the years while I was trying to simultaneously raise my kids, help raise my nieces, work, and be present for all of the extra things—some joyful, some difficult—that life had to offer. All these years, I have felt a strong desire to tell my story and share the stories of my beloved trans, nonbinary, and gender-expansive community. I also wanted to create something that those who come after us can hold in their hands and use to find some of what they might be looking for.

There are a few contributors from that initial attempt whom I was not able to reach in preparing for this publication, whose beautiful stories deserve to be read. I offer a sincere and deep apology to those authors and hope I will hear from them so that their stories can be included if there is a subsequent edition. I also want to acknowledge all the many people for whom it wasn't possible (or desirable) to contribute.

While writing this, I traveled to Salt Lake City, where I grew up, to be with my mom as she was nearing the end of her life. One morning I told her about the four deer I had seen earlier in the day. She said, "I love deer. Have I told you about the deer when I was pregnant with you?" I said that she had, but that I wanted to hear it again. In truth, I only remembered a ghostly wisp of the story, and I was hungry for stories from her to hold on to, ever more hungry as time with her thinned.

When my mom was pregnant with me, she was on a hike with my dad and some friends. She stayed back a bit, and while they were up ahead, she was having a solo moment of wonder in the beauty of nature and a deer just walked up to her! They took each other in. My mom said to me, "So that's why you're such a dear! But really, it was an amazing moment, and it made a big impression on me. Deer are very special to me."

Pregnancy stories are stories from thresholds, from times when we are undergoing change, when life might or might not come to be; they are stories as old as time, and yet each is unique.

Several years ago, a cis woman I am in community with took me up on an offer to talk with her about my experience as a trans person. She had a young person in her life who was transitioning, and she wanted to learn more about how to be supportive. She was surprised when I told her I love being trans. I think she expected to hear about hardship, but not about what a joy it is to live in my own intentional gender and to be a member of the trans community. Being part of this project has deepened my trans joy—reflecting on my own experience, learning and sharing the stories of others, and feeling the gift of enthusiastic support from friends, family, and allies.

This book comes forth during a period of rapid change. In many countries, journalists, health care providers, reproductive rights activists, and people speaking of pregnancy in general have begun to widely use the term "pregnant people" instead of "pregnant women." In my world, this is most obvious when I'm watching the news and Amy Goodman or one of her guests says "pregnant people." When I hear this, I grin, feeling like there's space for me and my family. This shift to more inclusive language is not universal, but to me it feels like an extraordinary leap from twenty years ago when I started this journey. Despite attacks from the right, intersectional feminism and critical race theory are gaining more widespread traction, helping us understand and describe where we are today and where we have come from.

Some of us have become midwives, doulas, doctors, and many other types of professionals who provide pregnancy-specific care and support. Now we have research studies, guides for practitioners, online groups, and a variety of other resources. There's even a masc pregnant person as part of the standard emoji set. And we have books! *Seahorses* joins several autobiographies and children's books about trans, nonbinary, and gender-expansive pregnancy—and you should read them all.

There is so much evidence that we exist! This is not small. This is the result of generations of activism by and for trans, nonbinary, and gender-expansive people and our allies. This is also the result of generations of activism by feminists and reproductive rights advocates. I saw these two worlds come together in 2015, when Birth for Every Body responded to an open letter to the Midwives Alliance of North America (MANA) from midwives who were fighting against gender-inclusive language.[1] I wept reading the response, seeing all those names of birth workers and others, signed in support of people like me, families like mine. I was deeply moved by how many people signed. I was delighted to see my midwife's name.

In 2024, the Utah State Legislature ("righteouslature" if you ask my lefty dad) made it illegal for trans people to use the appropriate restrooms, and because I generally pass for male, I would feel rude (and unsafe) using the women's.[2] I've been flying between Salt Lake and Seattle a lot lately because of my mom's health. The "family" bathroom in the Salt Lake airport has a transgender symbol on the sign, all official: raised up and frosted white, right below the family holding hands. It feels like a protest against Utah's regressive policies. I silently thank whoever chose that sign. (Were they sneaky? Did they fight for it? How did this happen?) At the Seattle airport, they recently installed a big gender-neutral bathroom with multiple stalls and sinks. It's bright and modern, and it doesn't seem to bother anyone.

These are the times we are in. We are visible, welcomed, sometimes made uncomfortably visible by how welcomed we are, and also losing the right to pee, or to change our babies' diapers, or to take medicine in private. The rhetoric of inclusion feels good to me, yet I also know that my rights are subject to cultural whims and the currency of power.

We are also in a time of unprecedented attacks on trans and nonbinary people and our rights. We are being invoked in campaigns of scare tactics by fascist far-right leaders and political movements.[3] Creating fear of us creates power for others. They cast us as a formidable threat because we are coming into power with those around us. We strengthen and are strengthened by the families, communities, and movements we are part of. To me, this feels like love. Love for ourselves and each other. This is the good stuff, and it's a damn shame that our liberation is being spun in ways that harm us.

A few of these politicians might be driven by a genuine, albeit misguided, crusade against us, but it seems most merely offer us up as part of a package—along with abortion, gun control, and immigration—that gets blood boiling in their base. Once they're in office, they often keep up with those hot items, but their real work is in removing limits to the aggregation of wealth and power and disassembling hard-won protections for regular people, unions, the environment, and our democracy. We are a pawn, and we are a useful pawn because we are so much more visible now. Even though anti-trans legislation isn't grounded in a real threat we pose, it still harms us in real ways.

Reproductive rights are also under attack in the United States. Combined with disproportionate and shocking pregnancy-related mortality rates for Black people, this means that Black people of all genders are forced into life-threatening pregnancies by legislative decree.

Outside of the US, trans, nonbinary, and gender-expansive people are also experiencing both unprecedented visibility and acceptance and unprecedented violence and legal threats. Internationally, we are thrown under the bus along with Indigenous people, women and girls, LGB folks, the environment, religious minorities, refugees and asylum seekers, people with disabilities, workers and unions, and more. We are in good company, and we are increasingly part of coalitions working to fight for the rights of everyone.

Most of this book was written on occupied land, during a time of wars, mass incarceration, climate crisis, ethnic cleansing, and genocide. May seahorse parents, all pregnant people, all people, and all beings live in safety, peace, and liberation. May our children thrive.

The SisterSong Women of Color Reproductive Justice Collective tells us that reproductive justice is "the human right to maintain personal bodily autonomy, have children, not have children, and parent the children we have in safe and sustainable communities."[4] I pray for more ceasefires than there are guns and bombs. I also want to recognize the additional impact that every injustice has on people who are pregnant, or want to be, or want not to be—people migrating under perilous conditions often do not have access to even basic medical care, let alone reproductive health care. Food insecurity takes away reproductive choice, housing insecurity takes away reproductive choice, racism and ableism take away reproductive choice, religious oppression takes away reproductive choice, and exploitative labor conditions take away reproductive choice. We are also in a time of widespread compulsory parenthood—most straight cis people are expected to have children, whether or not they really want to, another affront to reproductive choice.

In some places, sterilization has been required as a condition for accessing legal and medical transition. No one should ever have to choose between transition and the ability to reproduce. Sterilization that is forced or otherwise coerced is a violation of our bodily autonomy and a paternalistic attempt to limit and define the lives of trans people, our families, and our communities. It is a violence against transfeminine people, transmasculine people, and siblings of all genders who seek legal or medical transition.

Genocide, attacks on reproductive autonomy, forcing trans people (especially trans kids) into boxes—inside all of this, a tender thing is happening, a powerful thing. We are here. We have always been here, and we will always be here. Now is a time of chaos and fear, and also we are building beautiful alternatives. For some of us, creating a safe space in our bodies to nurture life is an act of resistance, and for others it is simply an act of love. For some of us, not being pregnant is a choice that can't be taken for granted. Some of us have weathered devastating loss, and some of us are still striving to become pregnant.

In *Testo Junkie,* Paul Preciado introduced the idea of the "techno body," the modern body that is constructed intentionally by the self and the social and commercial forces of the pharmaceutical, pornographic, and technological era. People now are using hormones and changing our bodies in ways that are sanctioned or unsanctioned. Bodies and social expectations of bodies are altered by the synthetic estrogen and testosterone many people use for many different reasons, as well as by the procedures by which we permanently or temporarily alter our bodies. We pick and choose our chemistry and anatomy and sex and gender in the presence of forces that profit from certain choices and thus aim to control our choices about chemistry and anatomy and sex and gender. It has been normal in our culture for cis people—and is increasingly normal for trans people—to (purchase and) take hormones by which we alter our capacity to reproduce, and of course it has been normal to reproduce, by which we alter our capacity to take hormones.

If we assume, for a moment, that sex and gender are two different things, like hardware and software, the sex of pregnancy can be something altogether different than "vagina" or "penis," "innie" or "outie." The sex of pregnancy can also be "other," "occupied," and "under construction." The organs become another dimension, a hideout, a workshop, a laboratory, a place where flesh and anticipation and ancestry and love churn into a person, or sometimes a place where something is amiss. Hormones bathed my cells in pregnancy, a wholly different chemistry than I'd had before or would have when I started taking testosterone after weaning my second child. Certainly not all trans, nonbinary, and gender-expansive people have the same hormonal journey or identify the sex of their pregnant bodies this way, but many of us invite a different layer of inquiry to what it means to be in our bodies, and in our genders, as we experience pregnancy. I believe this kind of intentional inquiry is one of our great gifts—for ourselves, and for cis people who want to dive in and explore the worlds of their own genders, bodies, relationships, and families.

Some people want us to disappear, some welcome us to assimilate like we are just the same as everyone else, and many celebrate our unique selves, pregnancies, and families. We and our children deserve equitable treatment, as well as acknowledgment that our paths and our families are different. We are gems. Our babies are miracles. Our families are revolutionary. Our troubles are both mundane and exceptional. Our bodies, which hold the capacity to create life, are beautiful.

We cannot exist in our own bubbles, because there are not enough of us, so we are naturally bridge builders. We are wisdom keepers, change makers, life givers, people who fuck up and keep going forward. We are allies who learn from our allies. Through our experiences with pregnancy and beyond, we are in communion with the next generation—even when that does not mean raising them.

I would like to honor Lili Elbe, a Danish transgender painter who died in 1931 from complications after an attempted uterus transplant. Ms. Elbe's dream of carrying and birthing a child is still not available to trans women or many of our other trans, nonbinary, and gender-expansive siblings. May we carry their dreams as our own until pregnancy is possible for everyone.

There is no real way to put down in words the miracles and heartaches of pregnancy, but it is one of life's greatest nexus points. How do we arrive as people with marginalized gender experiences? What do we discover at the intersections of our multiple identities? Who are we in our families and communities? Who are we in the world of pregnancy and birth, abortion and miscarriage?

This book is inspired by love for trans, nonbinary, and gender-expansive people and our families, and by the transcendent love I learned from my children, starting before I was pregnant with them. May you, dear reader, find tender threads weaving your story with ours and sparkles of life's infinite diversity.

Notes

1 Disappointingly, the open letter was signed by Ina May Gaskin, who deserves flowers for revolutionizing pregnancy and birth care in the US, which has benefited people of all genders, whether she likes it or not. The Birth for Every Body response can be found at: http://www.birthforeverybody.org/response-to-open-letter.

2 I, like many other people, believed that the law was broader in scope than it actually is. In fact, HB 257 primarily impacts people trying to access bathrooms, changing rooms, and locker rooms in K–12 public schools and changing facilities in government-owned buildings. These laws have a chilling effect that reaches beyond what they actually regulate, which, arguably, is the point.

3 For more on this, listen to the podcast *The Anti-Trans Hate Machine* by Imara Jones, of TransLash Media: https://translash.org/projects/the-anti-trans-hate-machine.

4 "Reproductive Justice," SisterSong, accessed April 28, 2025, https://www.sistersong.net/reproductive-justice.

S. Aakash Kishore

The Morning After

The morning after I gave birth to my firstborn, I sat at the edge of the hospital bed staring into their bassinet. Fourteen hours prior, I was still pregnant; now I was empty. Numb. I knew I couldn't stay in this room forever, and yet I couldn't bring myself to leave. So I just stared at my baby. They looked so different, their tiny body already succumbing to the ways that death changes things.

Ami was on the phone with the funeral home making arrangements for Sanchal's cremation. Overhearing that a backlog of work due to COVID-related deaths would delay us by several weeks, I reasoned that the gods would not hold us to the usual prescriptions of when to release the ashes. I'd entered this room on a Monday, three centimeters dilated and 80 percent effaced after finding blood in the toilet, with the hope that my cervix would stabilize enough to allow for the placement of an emergency cerclage. It didn't. By Tuesday morning, I was experiencing mild contractions and facing the reality of giving birth at twenty-one weeks to a baby whose lungs hadn't yet matured enough to survive outside my womb. I gave birth to Sanchal Thangamani en caul that evening, in as much fearless freedom as I could muster. Ami and I took turns holding them to our bare chests, my birth center midwife, Olivia, serving as a witness to the moment we became parents. Then I hemorrhaged. As I bled for four hours, the hospital staff was sparse, leaving Olivia to change out the chucks pads as I shook violently from a bone-deep cold despite the mountain of heated blankets she had diligently arranged for me. A little after midnight, the attending physician finally performed a D&C (dilation and curettage) to remove the bits of Sanchal's placenta that were still clinging to my uterus. Now I was here, tracing familiar contours on the face of my lifeless child, trying to sear each miniscule detail into my memory, and waiting for something to guide my next move.

If you'd asked her at the time, Ami would have told you I had a joyful pregnancy; I didn't. The elated disbelief of that second line appearing on the dipstick in early July after my first and only sperm exposure quickly slammed into the reality of my supposed gender transgressions. At work that morning, no less than three colleagues commented on how much weight I'd lost since January, pinching my sides and grabbing my shrunken biceps to prove their point. When I called to schedule my first ultrasound a few weeks later, the receptionist asked if I was calling on behalf of my wife. I told my parents I was pregnant toward the end of week eight. They're both scientists, but they had a lot of questions about how the pregnancy came to be. My mom couldn't wrap her mind around the fact that Ami had no desire to gestate a child and that I did. She wondered what restroom I was going to use now. My dad couldn't grasp why being trans and pregnant at the height of the pandemic made me unwilling to make plans to fly back to the Midwest for Thanksgiving. When we called Ami's parents to tell them a week later, her mom said nothing; her dad tried to hang up, and when he couldn't, he walked out of the room.

For her part, Ami was determined to do my pregnancy right, so she took to feeding our embryo the most nutrition-packed foods, getting frequently frustrated and offended when my body was less than willing to let me eat them. She whipped up a giant batch of white bean and parsley hummus, tried to feed me every bitter green from our garden, and rebuffed my carb cravings with warnings about juvenile diabetes. Afraid of losing herself to parenthood, she wanted us to do all we could to make memories before the baby came, so I spent much of my first trimester under an unrelenting summer sun doing my very best to participate. We tried to do what we would normally do, and I didn't know how to say no (except to the white bean hummus; I still can't talk about it).

As my pregnancy progressed, the mounting microaggressions began to drain me, and Ami was not prepared to witness—let alone support me through—that kind of pain. Her fierce love twisted into a gnawing anxiety that came out unpredictably sideways.

"Can we finish the garage?" she asked as we lay in bed one night. "I think I'll live out there in the first few years. I don't want to lose myself caring for this baby." A heaviness lodged itself in my throat as I wove my right arm under her pillow to wrap her shoulders in an embrace. I breathed what little breath I could find into my womb, imagining it shielding the tiny growing being inside me.

"If that's what you think you need, let's find a contractor."

"What if I end up leaving you?" she asked a few minutes later, through soft sobs. I stroked her hair, wiped tears from each cheek.

"I want you to do what you need to do to be happy," I told her solidly, my own safety and security crumbling away beneath me. Half a year earlier, when I was just stopping the testosterone I'd taken for twelve years and quickly feeling bits of my affirmed self destabilize, she'd held both my hands in hers and told me with a wholehearted earnestness that she would support me through everything our journey to parenthood might entail. Now that I was actually pregnant, was she having second thoughts? I could feel the bottom falling out as I struggled to reconcile her acts of care with her words of abandonment, and I quietly prepared myself to raise our child on my own.

That Tuesday in November, as I lay in the hospital bed feeling helpless in my body and expectantly waiting for my worst nightmare to be realized, I actually searched Ami's face for signs of relief. "I want to try for another child," I told her, unsure whether I'd catch a glint of hesitation in her eyes. When she nodded in agreement, I found myself both grateful and resentful. *How can she so easily agree when she seemed ready to abandon the baby we were about to lose?* But after it was all said and done, after an intense and beautiful birth, after saying hello and goodbye to our sweet Sanchal, after the bleeding and the D&C and waking to my own voice crying out desperately for my baby, Ami and I found we only had each other. On Wednesday morning, she helped me to the hospital bathroom so I could shower, standing by as I scrubbed at the blood-encrusted hairs of my thighs: the washcloth, the streams down my shins, and the pool around the drain all the same ruddy hue. When the bag was packed and the calls were made, when the papers were signed and I had wept over every surface in that room, we finally left without our baby and stepped out into the loneliest winter of our lives.

Everything inside our front door seemed confused by our return. I examined the stupid blue sofa. A bag of avocados sat useless on the counter. *Braiding Sweetgrass* lay expectantly on the bedroom nightstand, a small slip of paper marking where we'd left off family story time the night before it all unraveled. Nothing here knew what to do with us anymore. I stripped the beds. I pulled every blanket and pillow I could find into the middle of the living room floor, layering them one on top of the other, but it was wrong. I pulled them apart and layered again. And again. And again, until I collapsed in exhaustion. We ate soup. Ami turned on an episode of *Star Trek: Voyager* to fill the hollow of our home, and we slept until the afternoon turned over to evening.

Olivia came over twice in that first week. She sat with us on the blankets for hours. I asked her what happened, and she told me about the beauty of Sanchal's birth, about the attending physician's avoidant discomfort, how the doctor had administered fentanyl against my wishes and joked about needing my eyes to roll back in my head before entering my body and then dismissed Olivia's efforts to give me the agency to slow down. She didn't know why they'd let me bleed so long. We all cried together. She let there be long silences between my words. Or no words at all.

Nearly everyone in our community seemed to disappear into the dark wet of the holidays in the Pacific Northwest with the false belief that time and their silence would magically heal me. Us. Despite her own shocked grief, Ami made sure we ate every day. She set alarms on her phone to remind me to shower and pee.

"No one has asked me about suicidal ideation," I confessed in the last minutes of a video appointment with Olivia in late November.

"*Are* you experiencing suicidal ideation?" she asked earnestly.

I told her that the days were a series of seconds in which my body contorted its way through the memory of what happened. I said that if I slept at night I'd dream of the hospital, of bleeding, of losing my baby over and over again until I'd wake in a tangle of terror and tears. I told her that if I didn't sleep, I'd be inundated for hours with guilt, shame, and insistent images of my own death by hanging. I hated this useless body that had failed to hold Sanchal but was trapping me now. And I hated myself for having these thoughts about a body that had sacrificed so much and was still pulsing with the cells of my precious child.

Olivia helped me make a schedule to get through the days. I used it as my planner, diligently building checklists to pass the hours, then days, then months. I used it to track my sleep, my nightmares, my moods. After trying and failing to connect with multiple therapists, I titrated my own stimulus-response protocol to help me return to the bed at night and my own exposure hierarchy to help me venture out of the house during the day.

Saying goodbye to Olivia in our final appointment one snowy December afternoon felt like saying goodbye to Sanchal all over again. Memories of my pregnancy stuck to the corners of the birth center clinic. Upstairs was a room with a tub and a bed where my baby and I were supposed to meet but neither of us would ever see. Yet, that night at the hospital, Olivia had cradled Sanchal's tiny body in her arms when I'd offered them to her, gently pulling the receiving blanket down from their chin to fully take in their features. Olivia alone knew these fragments of me I could no longer fit into my old life. Still, it was unfair of me to burden her with this connection simply because I couldn't bear the thought of letting go. Perhaps she sensed my struggle; as we parted, she told me I could still text her. I said I wouldn't. I wasn't her problem anymore. She texted me the next morning instead.

Nothing was easy as I tried to heal myself enough to be ready to call in a second baby. Friends left. They literally packed up, moved out of our home, and didn't look back. The provider who helped us conceive Sanchal ghosted us. Every interaction hurt, and being alone with my thoughts was terrifying. Two weeks after my last visit to the birth center, I had my first sips of alcohol in months, ushered Ami off to bed, and wrapped a cord around my neck. As the pressure built in my head, I realized how unsurvivable it would be for Ami to find me here in the morning. I let go and was flooded with a deep, deep shame. I berated myself for setting such a poor example for my dead child. The urge didn't go away. It persisted, it looped, it begged and cajoled me for hours upon hours, nearly every night and often in the day.

Conceiving again was a struggle. I didn't have issues with fertility; I had issues with accessing trans-affirming and trauma-informed care. In my February and March cycles, I was so desperate for help with getting sperm inside me that I allowed an unsafe person to have access to my home, my family, and my body. I was left catatonic, fatigued, and broken. The act of repeatedly saying yes to someone who was inside me, out of fear of retaliation, undid what little trust I had begun to find in myself after my body failed to hold my first child. I was afraid to be touched, because I didn't believe in my own ability to say no, or that others would respect my boundaries. But when my LH (luteinizing hormone) peaked in April, I didn't have to deal with anyone but Olivia, who helped me practice safe touch in the days ahead and then cut short her ski trip, performing her very first IUI (intrauterine insemination) to help us make a baby.

I learned I was pregnant again on Mother's Day. Ami and I decided to keep this pregnancy to ourselves for as long as possible. It was too much last time to manage other people's projections, biases, and even hopes, and it was too much now to find grace for the inevitable missteps of what people would say or do about a pregnancy in the wake of loss. So we were on our own. At first, it was really beautiful. We had a chance to do things on our terms and with the insights we had gained from my first pregnancy. We still made memories, but we also made plenty of time for rest. I voiced cravings and Ami tended to them. Neither of us worried about how many bitter greens I ate, and every day we wrote little notes to Sanchal and the new life inside me. But as I made my way into the second trimester, old patterns reemerged.

Ami still hadn't prepared herself for the contorted stretching of embodied realities that it was for me to be trans and pregnant again after losing a child. She saw how it drained me to combat transphobia and erasure in every appointment, to beg to be treated with dignity while also somehow holding a sacred pocket for Sanchal and the little being we were getting to know in utero. She was angry at the systems that refused to see our family and angry at herself for not somehow having more skills to fight for us, but on most days that anger was expressed toward me. She needed respite, and as the halfway point of pregnancy approached, we agreed she should get away for a few days.

Olivia accompanied me to my anatomy scan—the one in which Ami and I had learned in my first pregnancy that my cervix might be shortening. She held my hand while we watched my baby kick, punch, and flip around on the monitor, perfectly Sanchal-sized but an energy all their own. We got good news—my cervix was long and strong, and the cerclage we'd had placed at the end of week twelve was still holding. The baby was healthy. Olivia exchanged information with the perinatologist about how to support the out-of-hospital birth that suddenly seemed within reach.

I expected to feel relieved, but it wasn't fair. The treetops blurred behind the grief pooling in my eyes as Olivia drove me back from the hospital. I had no words for her, just a collapsing feeling in my womb as I fruitlessly reached across timelines and prognoses to try to save both my children. I made it from her car to the house, where I slid down on the entryway doormat and cried for hours. When Ami returned the next day on the threshold of week twenty-one, she found me nonverbal and working the memory of Sanchal's last hours through my body. Everything from this point forward would be brand new, and I hated leaving Sanchal behind again.

"I don't want to be here," Ami blurted out a few days later as we returned home from our morning walk. "I wish I'd said no to you getting pregnant. I wish I'd said no to trying again after we lost Sanchal."

I stared at her, backlit in the doorway, as I braced myself on the counter across the room. She had been cold and disinterested since her return, leaving me to agonize over a schism that she insisted wasn't there. Here, finally, was the honest truth.

"Thank you for finally saying it." I felt conscious of my voice, how it was deep and solid through the echoing splat of tears hitting the wood floor. I rubbed the small pools into the dark grain with the toe of my sock. I listened for the *Wait, I didn't mean it* that never came.

The home I had in Ami was gone. When we'd met sixteen years prior, during the summer when I'd first named myself, she gently caught each piece of me that I dared to speak. She was the first person with whom I felt seen, but now it seemed as though she wished to erase me, erase the child we'd already lost, erase the one I was working so hard to keep safe. How were we here again after she'd expressed so much regret about how her anxiety had shaped my first pregnancy?

I was alone at the house when I started spotting a few weeks later. *This isn't happening. This isn't happening. This isn't happening.* Ami was staying at a rental while I scrambled to find some foothold for partnership with the person who was supposed to be *my* person. My co-parent. I compartmentalized each piece of the journey from my bathroom to the hospital and back again: *That's the road, and this is the steering wheel. Parking garage. An elevator. Ultrasound goop. Olivia and Ami. I can't look at Ami. A speculum. It's all reassuring. No, I don't want Ami home. Underwear, pants, shoes. Find the car keys, the hallway, the car. That noise. What* is *that guttural moaning? Oh, it's me. Ignition. Everyone's speeding on the freeway tonight. Wait, I'm going forty.*

Ami returned with a clarity that she did want the life we'd been building together, but I struggled to reconcile her newfound certainty with her ongoing threats of abandonment. She really just wanted the old me back: a simplified, seemingly normative version of masculinity that would withstand the swells of her anxiety—someone I could never be again. We talked a lot and we cried a lot. I asked "why" so many times, knowing I wouldn't get a satisfactory answer. I longed for the unbridled joy I'd imagined for myself in this phase of being so obviously, delightfully, a pregnant man. Instead, I scoured our relationship for the finest threads of trust with which I might weave a new safety net. More and more, I needed to bring this baby to term. Labor would be my chance to work through every loss I'd endured in the last two years, and I needed it to be all my own.

My water broke at thirty-four weeks and one day. After burning her breakfast while rushing to cancel the flight she was supposed to board that morning, Olivia met Ami and me in the same room in which I'd been triaged ten weeks prior. As it became clear I'd need to give birth too early to another baby, I told myself that this time was different. There was a cerclage to be removed and a clock to race to avoid risk of infection, but in all likelihood this baby would get what Sanchal never got: a chance at life.

Ami and I set an altar for Sanchal in one corner of the hospital room. The cerclage removal proved to be the trickiest one the doctor had ever done, but contractions started soon after it was out, steadily building overnight without augmentation. We were all patient with this baby and with each other. The nurses brought in beds for Olivia and Ami. They took turns resting and offering counterpressure during contractions to support the baby's descent, gently massaging me between. I stopped noticing whose hands were whose as the night wore on, focusing only on my breath as I invited my body to change with each rising wave. My baby and I were so in sync that no one else seemed to notice as I transitioned stages of labor, my cervix fully dilating just as the doctors came to tell me I'd reached their cutoff window of twenty-four hours for my labor to progress. There was a panicked flurry as staff rushed in, expecting the birth and a neonatal resuscitation to follow quickly. Instead, it took four patient hours of slow and steady movement before Kaanan Olimani was born into Olivia's waiting hands, our perinatologist shielding my family against her colleagues so that Olivia could catch the first baby she'd helped conceive. Kaanan breathed all on their own, giving voice to Sanchal in their first cries as

Olivia climbed up and placed them on my belly. For ten minutes, the room disappeared as we wept together, Ami leaning over my shoulder to help stimulate Kaanan's back.

The morning after Kaanan was born, I awoke in the Mother and Baby Unit of the hospital, not a mother and without a baby in my room. A nurse entered, eyed me in the hospital bed, swollen and bleeding from the events of the previous day, then turned to Ami and asked her if she'd had her baby yet. I inched myself out of the unit and down to the NICU, where Kaanan was being monitored, and where I sat in a chair and held them for as long as my body could tolerate sitting. The microaggressions and erasures were immediate and constant. Even as I mustered what little energy I could to advocate for myself and my baby, the power of what I'd just done quickly slipped away, my failures to protect Sanchal, and now Kaanan, instead coming into full focus.

When Kaanan was discharged home a week after their birth, Ami and I held them in every room of the house. We took them to the kitchen, the bedroom. We wheeled their bassinet next to Sanchal's altar in the living room and placed their tiny body in its vast expanse. We held the simultaneous presence and absence of our babies in our home, one of a whole lifetime of firsts and concurrent should-have-beens.

Long after the seasons of these pregnancies and births have passed, the cells in my womb still reach for Sanchal in a way that floors me. I yearn for a sense of wholeness, knowing that even as I willingly stretch my love across dimensions daily, my family won't ever quite feel complete. One afternoon, Olivia sits with me at our altar, remembering Sanchal and everything we walked together to bring Kaanan earthside. As she holds me, I find myself in full surrender, each sob plumbing a deeper grief than the last for everything I've lost. When I've worn myself out, she pulls me closer and tells me something I need to hear: I didn't get the joyful, supported pregnancy I had envisioned, but I absolutely deserved it.

Tom

8.8.8
time just continues
You and I
neither starting nor stopping
love between two parts going forever
boat of two
the course set
then
wayward waterways
tik tok
time to take stock
questioning:
boat of three?

Eight years feels like infinity, and the number, when turned on its side, becomes just that. My partner and I had been together for eight years before we seriously talked about kids. During that time, our weekdays were filled with ten-hour workdays and a bottle of wine each night regardless whether we were working the next day. We prepared luxurious dinners that could cost someone a week of their salary. We curated a network of friends who had decided that they were more interested in foraging for obscure wild mushrooms and VP careers than a life with children.

In eight years, I had built a community from those working in Seattle's tech industry, art scene, and health care but who for the most part were white, cisgender, straight liberals. I placed a lot of hope in this community of people. I planned for them to carry me through the toughest of situations that were yet to come. I'm bewildered now by the community I had built around me. I had no idea that postpartum depression, COVID, Asian hate crimes, and Trump were around the corner and would be my wake-up call, later making my values clearer. A more intentional path to building community has been clearer since all of those things happened. There were too many resources in my life before all of that, and it kept me from seeing what I needed to change.

When I asked myself whether I could have kids, the topics of racism, biracial identity, queerphobia, climate change, and all the systemic oppressions of the world were also brought up. I thought, *Is it irresponsible to bring up kids in such a messed-up world?* Barack Obama was president, the pandemic had not happened yet, I had a steady job, and my parents were relatively healthy. However, any hope was shadowed by my inner doubt, which surfaced like a slowly rising tide, despite the positivity that I might have felt.

Flash of light
stars and dust made of magic
one wizard and one magician
then there you were.
Can this be?
I concocted this spell
yet I don't have the incantation memorized
where is the correct book of spells?
whispers wash over a flickering candle
Is it in my head?
Or is this just rustling of the grass inside
enchantments or
nature's unfolding

Pregnancy is an act of faith with one's body, and the magic that happens during and after is wondrous and frightening. As a child, I didn't pay too much attention to my body. I felt ashamed of and embarrassed by it; it wasn't meant to possess the magic of mothering, creating, or birthing a child. As a young person, I saw wonder and delight in the external things around me, such as the Easy-Bake Oven, a toy that magically produces baked goods. As a kid, I didn't know that the Easy-Bake was plugged in to get hot. I just thought you'd stick in raw dough and it would come out baked, like some form of wizardry. Also, it was magical how all the kids who had the toy were so pleased by their creation, regardless of how it looked or tasted. I imagined the boastful glee of underbaked and oversprinkled delights. Why and how were they so happy? This was the true magic.

Then, *poof*, a cloud of smoke appeared and in less than a year after stopping the pill, there I was, with a child on the way. The easiness and magical quality of the whole experience was quickly overtaken by a period of searching for my pregnancy euphoria. I am not sure where I got this idea, but I presumed it to be real. You know, the joyous elation that you see in the faces of those pregnant on social media or those on the Easy-Bake commercials? Instead of happiness, I was anxious and doubtful that the "magic" would work. I didn't say it out loud. I kept it to myself. I spoke incantations like, "Oh yes, the easiest pregnancy ever!" instead of the fire and brimstone that was simmering in my mind that would have scared the pants off of anyone. I didn't allow myself to go down into that black cauldron of doubt. Instead, I stuffed it away like the clothes I wouldn't wear for the next nine months.

In part, I could not fathom that I was conjuring a human inside of my belly. *Yeach*, I often thought to myself. I barely could stomach the ultrasound or the thought of hearing the heartbeat, when I knew these were all "supposed to be" such sweet and tender moments. I felt that they were more science fiction than real life. Even more disconcerting was that no one else thought that this was abnormal, a being living inside your stomach and feeding off of you. I was not a mother, I was a host. My hair and skin transformed: *Is this natural? If it's so natural, why aren't more pregnant people freaking out right now?*

I worked in human resources at a hospital while I was pregnant, which was the least mystical place one could work. Some might see the work of doctors quite the opposite, but it is a bit sterile when you work behind the scenes. I didn't tell many people about my pregnancy, including my coworkers. When I finally did let them know, I had comments like, "I knew you were pregnant because you started walking funny," and, "I noticed you started to have a cute little pooch." Everyone felt at liberty to talk freely about my body and how I looked. If they weren't commenting about their own pregnancy experiences, they were commenting on what mine would be like. One day, my coworker who was a parent said, "You look great for being in your third trimester." I couldn't tell if this was a compliment or something else entirely. Meanwhile, I was trying to run away from my body. If I had a potion of invisibility, I would have taken it in a heartbeat. Some looked at me with sadness, others with delight, and some were curious. The othering that I felt during pregnancy felt familiar. It was how I had felt growing up Japanese in a mostly white school and neighborhood. It was how I had felt othered when I was called "Jap" in school or when people said, "Your English is so good!"

My partner and I waited for things to happen when I came close to my due date. Time slowed as if a magic wand had cursed us. Two days turned into four, which turned into eight. The doctor mentioned inducing if I didn't have any contractions in the next day or so. The tide of worry resurfaced, but now it was spoken out loud. The magician's smoke cleared, and what appeared were many hours of pain, drug-induced delirium, and exhausting labor that felt like days. As I was lying in the hospital bed, the doctor said the phrase "heartbeat troubles" and something about the umbilical cord rusting away. In my delusion, I imagined a rusty wire running from me to the baby inside my belly. "We waited as long as we could, it's time." My doctor was implying that a C-section was the best decision at the time, and I agreed with her. The illusions of a natural childbirth faded, and the metamorphosis was about to begin. I felt scared and relieved, but instead of being an onlooker to a wondrous trick, I suddenly became the magician's assistant. The person that lies down inside a body-sized box, smiling and trying not to freak out. Then, without regard, the magician saws me in half.

The clock's ticks are loud
and carry across the silence of our house.
In my head, the hands of time knocking back and forth
shadows overwhelm my soul in those hours, minutes, and seconds
Is it tomorrow yet?
What month is it?
What day?

After the baby was born, the constant feeding, diapering, sleep-supporting, and playing caused me to lose track of time. The days felt like forever. Had time actually stopped? I recall looking at the clock, 9:05 a.m., and wondering when my partner was coming home. I had only been on my own since 8:30 that morning. It felt like a lifetime to live through a day, and I continued to become even more disconnected to my body after the magician's trick on the operating table. I woke up each morning feeling less of myself.

Breastfeeding was particularly hard. It is common after C-sections that, due to the trauma to the body, breast milk does not arrive. I stumbled on that fact much later and only after countless hours sitting hooked up to a breast pump. Time just slipped away. I watched the minutes and seconds go by on the timer, waiting for the pumping session to end. "This isn't right," I kept saying to myself after extracting a tablespoon of milk at a time. Being hooked up to a pump was infuriating and dehumanizing. Luckily my partner and I decided to start formula feeding early. He felt a deeper connection and contribution to those late-night and early-morning bottle feedings. However, the articles and parent blogs didn't say anything about this feeling that seethed inside of me during those pointless days of pumping. My anger turned toward the world's expectations of breastfeeding and pumping, which weren't possible for me.

If I can't breastfeed, does that make me less female or less of a mother? I felt more like a father in the binary parenting spectrum. Isn't there something else that I can be? All of this questioning was hard to articulate back then. Gender roles smacked me in the face when it came to household chores, caretaking, and working outside the home. My mothering quickly reverted back to my upbringing by my own mother. She was a third-generation Japanese American during the 1950s who valued working hard and saving money, more than you will ever need. Being safe and not doing anything risky. Then my parenting morphed into a mix of early feminist theory and rebellious teenage punk rock. I was very confused and tormented by this disparate imprinting on my parenting. My body entered a state of slumber, and my passions in curating art, writing, gardening, and socializing became obsolete. Who was I, if not those things? My entire foundation went missing. I felt like I was drifting out to sea.

I can't go back. I remember standing in the shower wishing that I didn't have to come out of the safety and aloneness that I deeply felt. I didn't know how long I'd been standing there and only knew I had to get out when the water started turning cold. In that time, I would go to another planet, visit a place where I didn't have parenting responsibilities or the social pressures of being a mother. I wondered if I had made a mistake. In those hours of standing there, alone, suicidal thoughts ran over me like the water I stood beneath, but the thoughts didn't wash away into the drain like I wanted them to. They stayed. Later, I learned the term *derealization*, a condition when you feel that you're observing yourself from outside your body or that the things around you aren't real. Sometimes it feels as if you are living in a dream or in a movie. Where did I go? My heart was searching, a restless unsettledness that didn't subside.

"Don't you want to drive to places?" my mother-in-law inquired when I mentioned I wasn't getting out much. I didn't really understand her question. She was asking in her gentle way if I needed any help. I think there had been private conversations about my mental health between my partner and her, and she was reaching out for a visit on a sunny afternoon. I remember looking down at the ground, work gloves covered in dirt, my newborn in a carrier at my side, and realizing I was weeding a part of the garden that didn't need it. She cared, but she didn't have an answer. She may have been wise, but she had no idea what was going on inside of me. She had sympathetic words, but she couldn't tell me to go to a therapist. She had raised two children of her own, one of whom is my partner. She could not have told me what I would have experienced after the birth of my child and that my core would be shaken so much that I wouldn't know myself anymore.

Restarting life without a manual
nothing seemed to work until
I laid my wristwatch on the kitchen table
tenderly, I held the watch face up cradling it in my hand
the watch's face looking back at me
I'm so far removed from you, it said, we'll never be one again.
Pull out the watch's stem a voice from my past called out
Use your thumb and index finger slowly and thoughtfully
Wind your watch's stem lovingly the tree whispered
Be careful with your watch's components, never shove or force.
Then like the softness of the wind,
barely audible at times or seen clearly
the watch's hands restarted.

I looked at my watch because I wanted to be on time for my first therapy session. I remember completing a form at the hospital as part of my check-in. I was by myself, alone with my thoughts and body, a rare occurrence. My partner and newborn were together enjoying the sunshine while the darkness loomed in my heart as I waited for my appointment. The survey asked about depression levels and my sexual activity and pleasure. I hung on the words *sex* and *pleasure*, which appeared blurry and felt watery in my head. I didn't know what those words meant. I remembered what they had meant before pregnancy, but now those memories felt hollow. The last few months of child-rearing had also seemed vacant of pleasure. After those sessions with the therapist and my peer counselors, I realized my sadness and anger stemmed from leaving so many of my identities behind.

In my first middle and high school relationships, I was attracted to and hooked up with girls and boys. Everyone in our circle practiced "open relationships." We didn't have the words or the agreements and consent or the poly community. There was a group of us, most of whom were bisexual; today I identify as pan-sexual. We were looking for freedom from the confines of our binary world, finding our voice in political activism, punk music, fighting for LGBTQ rights, and getting arrested for passing out condoms in high schools. The police and government represented control and power, and our open-relationships community was liberation from these confines. I remembered parts of myself and the community that raised me. I remembered what I valued and cared about was still true today.

Being non-binary is a tree that continues to grow, creating shade, food, and shelter. All of the elements needed to create a healing pathway forward: the shade for rest and reflection, the food to nurture and learn, and the shelter to weather the storm of the world's oppressions. The support and care from the queer community is a large, colorful, flowery evergreen bush that, as it continues to evolve, uplifts and inspires me so that I am able to just be me. I am more powerful in my body when I can express a gender that doesn't label or put me in a box. There is a regaining of control over not being one or the other parent in my relationship to my child because of my gender identity. There is a deeper closeness I feel with my child knowing that they see me as who I am most comfortable being in the world. Being non-binary is the balm to my hurt from the oppressions of sexism. It is the elixir that gives me fierceness and conviction when my voice goes silent. There are still overcast days, but being queer has freed me from so many sorrows and allowed me to take flight from the confines of a binary identity of motherhood.

J. Workman

Try-Again Time

The majority of my childhood photos are in a tattered Converse shoe box that is barely holding itself together. I've been carting it around from apartment to apartment for more than twenty years. I haven't gone through the photos in a long time, but while I was pregnant, one of those photos came out of the box to sit with me often. I am around six years old, standing in my grandparents' yard on Main Street in Waynesville, the antiques capital of Ohio. My favorite climbing tree has yet to be cut down, and I am in front of it, a silly grin for the camera spread across my face. I have the same bowl cut as most of the white boys in my kindergarten class, signaling its place in time like any good signature haircut does. My Aunt Lisa has a salon with four chairs where her garage used to be, and the slightly jagged cuts are attributed to my notorious inability to sit still in the chair, nothing to do with her skill. I am barefooted and shirtless, shoulders puffed up, hands on my back pushing my belly out. My orange shorts hitting just above the knees. I look proud.

As an adult, I often feel stuck in the thinking place. The leap from planning to action is a gulf so big it feels like I will surely die. I wish I could embody a do-or-die spirit when approaching big decisions, but somewhere along the line I internalized: *Do and die. Don't do—don't die.* I don't do many things that feel desperately necessary. I spend countless hours wallowing in the infinite space of indecision. By the time I am thirty-seven years old, there are two burning life decisions that still haven't been made, and though they are not innately in opposition, in my life they are on a collision course, the stakes of which get higher and higher with time: Start T or get pregnant?

I knew I wanted to be a parent from as early as I understood it as an option. The first role I ever tried on was big sibling, and it fit like a glove. I was charged with caring for my brother from an early age, and I took my job seriously: I fed him, played with him, bossed him around, brought him with me wherever I went. My first jobs were babysitting gigs, and childcare remained an important part of my life well into adulthood. I never had any doubt that I would be a parent—I just had no idea how it would happen.

By the time I turned eighteen, I had been inside of a hospital three times. The first time, I was two and a half years old, a sewing needle all but buried in my foot after a round of jumping on the couch against the warnings of my mother. The second time, a year later, I watched with wide eyes as my brother's body came careening into the world. The third time, fourteen-year-old me held my brother's warm hand as a doctor took him off life support and he took his last breath.

Much of my indecision about getting pregnant boiled down to a couple of core fears. I had already waited so long to transition. I thought, *If I wait longer, if I go in what feels like the other direction, what if I never make it back again?* I worried that I had already missed the chance to do both. It was already too late. I also worried about what my child would call me, and more importantly who would I be to them? How would other people see me in relation to my kid? How would I tell them that I am not my child's mother? What would I have to offer my child that is solid enough to stand on, to root in, to grow from? I went around and around with myself and these questions, worries, fears, and what-ifs for years, falling further into the well of indecision, looking for something to hold on to so I could climb out.

I went on a solo trip in the middle of nowhere. Being alone, away from everyone—the only way I know how to hear an answer loud enough to trust. I prayed and, on the way home, I gave my brother's ashes to the ocean. I had been holding on to my third of them, in the same cardboard box they came in, for nearly two decades. I returned from my trip with a feeling of possibility I hadn't felt in years. It was palpable and unexpected, less of a presence and more of an absence, a weight lifted, space for something new.

I come home with my mind made up, and not more than a month later, I am pregnant. I feel proud of my body for getting something right.

I am seasick for months. I sleep sitting up, and I dream I am stranded on a raft, ocean roiling around me. My partner, Esi, feeds me rice crackers in the middle of the night. Desperate attempts at staving off the sickness, at creating an equilibrium that I simply cannot find. My body grows and changes. No one seems to notice. I don't feel more feminine, more infused with some elusive essence of whatever it is to be a woman. I feel more connected to the little kid in that picture. I keep going back to it, trying to glean some wisdom from that little guy. What did he know then that I don't know now?

From the moment I find out I am pregnant, I know I will not be giving birth in a hospital. I will be at home, and our baby will be born there. These are not questions for me, not decisions that have to be mulled over and over again. I associate hospitals with death. I shut down when I am with doctors, even in the least vulnerable situations. Prior to trying to get pregnant, the last time I went to a doctor—for a routine checkup—she asked me what parts I had and said, "Sorry, I just have to ask so I know what to do." This is after I filled out the intake form, giving her the answer to her question. It appeared she was double-checking. Just to make sure. Her exact question was, "What parts do you have?" It spilled out of her mouth with no eye contact. I had trouble letting her examine my naked foot. In hindsight, I have empathy for her attempt, for her need for growth, her very human inability to be everything to everyone, but I'm not rolling the dice.

To have a home birth, everything needs to change. We upend our lives, move two hours north of the city we live in, rent a house overlooking the river, and contemplate the arrival of our new roommate. I find a midwife, and Esi starts the process of figuring out what we will need for a baby. This part is a mystery to me. Just the kind of chasm I cannot leap over. Faced with so many options, I decide we need nothing. Lucky for me, for our child, Esi takes the reins and makes sure we are prepared to welcome the child.

Birth brings out the jock in me. It starts with a sharp toss into the ocean, and it is sink or swim from the very first contraction. The contractions do not come with breaks like I have been told they will. Once I am there, in the plunging waves, my body takes over. I am strong. My thoughts swim far away from me. I am lighter. I am on my toes. My body knows exactly what to do. I get out of the way. The sensations are unimaginable. Nothing I can name. I endure. I am inside of every single moment until the end. I go blank. I am spent. I have left it all on the field, given it more than my all. In many ways, it feels like the pinnacle of my own masculinity. I come back to see our baby. She is in motion, being lifted up from the floor into my arms. Both of her big brown eyes are open wide. Esi cries with joy, her arms wrapped around me from behind. She takes the baby to a rocking chair on the other side of the room. The chair sways silently, the carpet underneath swallowing any sound. All I can hear is the baby's bleating. I bleed and bleed. I require stitches. I continue to bleed. I pass out. I come back and there is honey overwhelming my mouth. Someone put it in there. I have never tasted anything more repulsive. I pass out again. I come back. I hold the baby. She is more beautiful than I know how to handle. She is here now. Her name means "light of dawn." The sun is rising; the hardest part of her journey comes in the first moments of this new day, breaking open.

Soft light is beginning to bleed back into the sky from that familiar wound on the horizon, and I am holding the baby. The baby is crying. We have been lying in this bed together for enough hours to make a little more than two days if strung together tightly. Everything has loosened: my body, my mind, my grasp on time and form. Given the light, she must be going on two days old. I have not slept in the two days she has been here plus the ten hours it took to bring her.

I cannot close my eyes. Esi and the baby slept on and off throughout the night, but I could not. When I turned toward the baby, her tiny body that smelled like fire made my whole body buzz awake, vibrating with the newness of her presence. And when I turned away from her, I was convinced that it meant I didn't have what it takes to be a parent after all. What kind of parent needs to retract mere hours after they have met their baby for the first time? No, I would give her my full attention. I sat up. I lay back down. I curled my body around hers, so tiny that she fit perfectly inside the circle made from drawing my knees up to my chin. I marveled at her body, her human form on the outside now. I smelled her head full of fire. I listened to her strange sounds and arrhythmic breath.

I cannot close my eyes, because there, behind them, a moonless and beating world opens and envelops me. Takes me back to the place I had to pass through to get her. Maybe it was death's world. Or my own nightmares. Knobs protrude from holes, teeth gnash, the trees loom large and have eyes, snakes slither underfoot, everything swirls and howls and I am stuck there, in the threat, in the eye of the screaming. With my eyes open, I can see the sidewalk outside the window, the neighbors' houses, the Hudson River, the lavender blooms of the jacaranda tree. I can see my body, the baby's body, Esi's body, the three of us in this room, on this bed, in the flesh and freshness of it all. I can put some visual distance between me and the me who was, mere hours before, in the storm and the surrender.

Here I am, giving the baby my full attention, and she is still crying. Wailing. Ravenous. She is frantically gnawing at her arms, sucking her fingers, crying. Later versions of this scene will make us laugh until we cry, but now it is bone dry and desperate.

Esi sits next to me on the bed, trying to help us, trying to help me help the baby latch. I bring the baby's tiny mouth to the nipple, and she opens her baby bird mouth wider. Too small to lob her head, she meeps and beeps and cries and tries, but no dice. I try over and over again. We turn on a light, its brightness harsh and illuminating our struggle. I hold her head in the palm of my hand and push her toward the nipple again. Her tiny body thrashes, and her cries become more and more despairing.

The feeling inside me is a brand-new one. Never felt it before a day in my life. My breath has all been sucked out, and I am sure I will die for my inability to assuage the baby's cries. Day two of being a parent. *Unable to quell the cries of a child* scrawled on my tombstone. Everything in me tightening and tightening, like ratcheting on the bolts of a tire, cranking down the lid of an already too-tight jar. My own tears stream hot down my cheeks, melting into the pot of desperation we are making together.

Esi scoops the baby into her arms and whisks her away, singing softly to her and assuring me that a few moments away is what we don't know we need. When she brings her back, I try again. The trick the midwife taught us works this time. Cup the back of the head with a firm hand, tilt up the chin so the mouth falls open, and push her head onto the nipple until she starts to suck. This time she latches, and I feel that mounting need in her dissipate. I pop like a balloon, and we sink down, collapsing into the oxytocin exchange between us. She falls asleep and I fall quiet.

My two-and-a-half-year-old helps me make coffee almost every morning. It's one of our things. She climbs her ladder, joining me at sink height. I pour the beans in the grinder, and as soon as I place the lid on, her body strains up, arms reaching out, "BABA, BABA, that's my job!! I want to do the grinder."

"Of course, my love, I'm just getting it ready for you."

She relaxes a little and holds up her hand. "Which one is my thumb again?"

"You tell me!"

"Is it this one?" She holds up the thumb on her right hand proudly.

"Yes, that's it!" She presses down with her thumb, tongue out in a show of concentration, the grinder turning on and off like a record skipping, disjointed and unpracticed. Next comes the scooping. Some mornings she is seamless. Dipping into the ground coffee and coming up with a half-full scoop, carefully bringing it to the mouth of the filter and pouring it in without spilling a single shred of coffee. Other mornings, it is try-again time. Over and over again. "Oops, I spilled it, Baba. I spilled it ALLL OVER THE FLOOR! No worries," she says, before I can even step in to give her the reassurance she clearly doesn't need. "I'll try again!"

One of the books in her regular bedtime rotation is called *Try-Again Time*, and it has opened up a sky of possibility for her, given language to something so innate and intuitive to her toddler lifestyle. She applies it to everything. Spills, of course, make up a good portion of the everything. Spilled cup of water: TRY-AGAIN TIME. Spilled soup, juice, crayons, pee from the potty, rice, food and beverages of every stripe: TRY-AGAIN TIME! But we have other try-again times too. Experimental kick to my stomach during a diaper change: try-again time! Accidental fall off the back of the couch: try-again time! First attempt at putting on a shirt, buttoning a button, taking off pants, turning on the faucet, knowing when she needs to pee: TRY-AGAIN TIME.

For me, parenthood is one big try-again time. It is, possibly, the first time in my life when trying again is the only option. I cannot freeze. Everything is always in motion. My child always needs me. She is always growing, at dizzying rates. There is no pause button. I cannot hide parts of myself. It is too intimate. I make mistakes. All the time. All I can do is try again. All I can do is keep showing up. Bringing her into the world has forced me to finally catch up with myself. The first time in my life where I cannot hide. Even when only parts of me show up, I am all here.

Conversation: Personal Journeys

How did pregnancy change your relationship with your body or your gender?

Aakash Kishore: I'm still figuring this one out. In some ways, I feel more okay with the seeming contradictions within my body and with other people seeing those. I feel more confident exploring femme expression and more of a desire to do this—an active desire to not be read as cis/straight. For example, I used to try to minimize the curve of my waist and hips, but now I don't mind it and even at times dress to accentuate it. I used to feel a lot of fear (and shame?) about how care providers might interact with my body, and so I would avoid getting care, but I'm a lot more proactive with seeking that out now and with finding providers who treat my body right.

But I also struggle in my relationship with my body after losing my first child due to cervical insufficiency. My body still remembers the sensations of my baby slipping from me before they or I were ready, the helplessness and lack of control over what was happening to them and over what happened to me in the aftermath. I've been angry at and ashamed of my body for failing to keep my baby safe. As much as I wish and have tried so many different ways to move past or release those emotions, I believe I will always contend with them to some degree.

Simon Knaphus: This is a big question! I'm still figuring this one out too, and it's been a long time! One thing that became real for me when I was pregnant was that my body was part of a flow of life from before our human ancestors and going toward an unknowable future. My body's capacity to create life awed me. It felt so new and exciting, and, in a way, it was hard to believe that my body could create life, and in another way, I came to really understand that I was part of a bigger story of life on this planet. Since then, I have had a hysterectomy, and I ended up needing to do spiritual work—guided by a dear friend—around losing that significant organ. I didn't know going into it that I would need that; I figured I was done having babies, so it was just a bit of flesh hanging out in my body causing hormones and potentially harboring the same cancer my mother had. I also had mysterious back pain after that surgery that ended up being referred pain from internal scar tissue. Physical therapy and massage helped. This is my PSA to folks who get hysterectomies—keep an eye out for pain that may be caused by scar tissue! No one told me, and it took years to figure it out.

I didn't have top surgery until I knew I wasn't going to have more babies, which had been my plan all along. It was hard for me when my chest started growing during pregnancy, and I stopped wearing a binder about halfway through due to physical discomfort. Being able to make milk for my babies was worth it for me, but I know that isn't true for everyone. I went from hiding my chest as much as possible to mammal-feeding my babies in public, which was a big change! I'm grateful for the work of lactation activists who have made feeding babies in public something that, while not always accepted, is an openly declared right. I'm also grateful for my parents and the feminist punks and queer, disabled, sex worker, and fat activists who gave me great framework about my right to have a body and use it how I wanted without shame. It's not that I never had or have shame, but I knew that body shame is an oppressive outside force, not something wrong with me.

In a way, pregnancy was another transition for me—a transition in how I inhabited my body, moved through the world, envisioned the future. Transitioning to male in a way prepared me for transitioning to parent. I did also feel more masculine than before pregnancy in ways I didn't expect. Being pregnant affirmed my gender for me—I felt most at home in my gender when I found a male lane alongside female pregnant people but did not travel in the same lane, if that makes sense. I was fortunate to have a supportive community of women who were or had been pregnant who included me but didn't need me to be like them.

Pain changed for me. Having experienced pain that is part of a healthy process helped me understand another dimension of what pain can be, and learning to move through the pain of contractions before and during labor has taught me a lot about moving though other pain life has offered. Another body thing that comes to mind is that oxytocin rush feeling. I had definitely had tastes of that before being pregnant, but even after having top surgery I still get the sensation of milk letting down sometimes, like when I'm overcome by love for my kids, or occasionally when I see a tiny baby. The oxytocin is a chemical process, a body function, but it also has so much to do with who we are as a social species (and I imagine other mammals experience it too).

Amber Hickey: This is a tough one. I feel like I became more self-assured and vocal in my gender identity during my first pregnancy because I had to in order to avoid or respond to unintentional microaggressions when in public, at the hospital, etc. In the past, I have often felt like I am not queer enough to claim queerness (clearly, I am self-policing!). But I became a lot more comfortable in owning that part of my identity. I think it's also linked to the way I parent my kiddo. We didn't assign a gender at birth and are waiting for them to articulate their own identity. I still feel more comfortable advocating for them than for myself, but I'm definitely getting better at that too.

During both pregnancies, I've become more aware of my body's vulnerability, as well as impressed with what it can put up with. Before baby number one, I had never experienced chronic pain or any serious health issues. During and following that pregnancy, I have experienced: severe hip pain, strange skin issues, C-section scar pain, weakness in my core due to diastasis recti, and a still-new diagnosis of multiple sclerosis, which flared up about nine months after my first baby was born. It's been difficult, but I also feel relieved that I have found ways to feel pretty good and build a solid care network despite all the challenges.

Tom: This question is like a lingering leaf during the fall season: It hangs on and there will be a new leaf in its place the following year. I recently (February 2024) took a class called BIPOC Revolutionary Mothering with Aimee Suzara—I intentionally went with the idea of writing about my relationship to my body, but I was hesitant who might be there and what my classmates might start to say or assume about me. After the four weeks, I came away with a body manifesto that was fierce and tender about grief and healing related to being raised socially as female and the gender expectations and assumptions that were placed on me. My piece for *Seahorses* is the answer to this question, so I won't share too much—but ultimately it was my pregnancy and the birth process and the postpartum that solidified my relationship with my body and my values of honoring mine and others. I am so thankful for my young person who has gifted me with all this and has been my best ally ever since.

Kara Johnson Martone: My answer to this is layered and ever changing. One thing I notice is that my feelings about my body have shifted a lot since childbirth. I notice that the judgment toward myself that I carried before pregnancy has softened. My internal dialogue has shifted to a much kinder and neutral place. At times, I even find myself having appreciation for my curves and soft spots. My body feels like a soft and comforting place for my child to find comfort. Through this I have begun to realize that my body is a soft spot for me to return to as well.

One area that continues to cause discomfort is my C-section scar. I still have mixed and confusing feelings about that scar and what I went through to get it. I have learned a lot about the limits of my body and how I have often pushed myself beyond those limits. There is a lot of grief that I continue to process with that experience and with my body.

In terms of my gender, this is something that is always in flux. As my baby grows into a toddler, I notice others' perceptions of me more and more. It becomes clear what boxes people feel comfortable placing me in. There is a picture of who we are as a family and how we identify that will always be wrong. Coming to peace with that has allowed me to feel more freedom in the way I express my gender.

g k somers: I speak to this a bit in my piece, but I actually felt probably the most at home I ever have in my gender when I was pregnant. Being trans has been such a beautiful gift of freedom in my life—freedom from expectations, freedom from following a path that was written for me. I felt so incredibly gender expansive while pregnant, and I think there's this overarching narrative about trans people that dysphoria is going to look a certain way, which often pertains to this binary perspective of man/woman, and that's just not true for everyone. Yeah, sure, it can be true for some people, but I really want to believe that the more we own our diverse narratives, the less people will feel compelled to fit into binary structures and more free to just be their ever-evolving selves, no matter what that looks like.

Zillah Rose: Prior to having given birth, I always felt that though my gender dysphoria was complicated, I felt comfortable and liked myself even within that dysphoria.

When I chose to stay pregnant, I knew my body was going to morph and change and evolve to some new version of me. Despite that uncertainty, I was excited to be pregnant. I felt like I got to wear a drag pregnant belly and be this otherworldly magical being who got chosen to carry another life. How epic is that?! When my belly rounded so far out that I then had a built-in table while sitting on the couch . . . stellar. Every day I looked in the large bathroom mirror at work and repeatedly thought, *How could I be so lucky?* I, who always had loss after loss after loss, after giving up and now . . . now chosen by some cosmic intervention to be this something "new." New me, new life, new learning, new unlearning, new depleted tired and new never getting to sleep . . . heavy body, growing body, stretch marks body. I felt like my body was a poem written about love.

I rewatched my birthing video prior to writing this, with my child in my lap, who kept saying to me, "Look see, that's me, I was inside you and then I was born!" I need these moments to remind me now, in hindsight, oh that's right, I am so lucky that I chose to carry my child in this body that grieved the existence of gender dysphoria most of my life to now carry you, my sweet child, in my arms.

People often mistake me as my child's grandmother. The grandma comments do sting. Not because of my nearing elderly age or crone beauty, but because my body that used to say, "Hey, I am both [genders]," now says, "I may be someone's grandma because I have a socially labeled body shape of someone who gave birth, and generally that means woman." My internalized gender dysphoria and socially ingrained transphobia argues that because I look so much like X and less like Y, unless I go under the knife, I will stay like this, and forever incorrectly be called "mom" and "grandma." I no longer look in that mirror that once said, "Wow, just look at you, you amazing lucky person." I hope to change that . . .

I am still grateful I chose to grow my child in my womb. But who am I as a confident genderqueer person? I hope to find myself again.

Was your spirituality impacted by pregnancy? Was your pregnancy impacted by spirituality? Did spiritual practices play a part in your

experience of pregnancy? (If the word "spirituality" doesn't work for you here, please consider responding and sharing language that would include your experience.)

Aakash: Yes. So much yes to this. Although my spouse and I were both raised Hindu and would at times go through the general steps of a puja for various holidays, we hadn't deeply sat together in prayer or meditation until we started preparing for conception. I found myself in a place of grief after coming off T and getting reacquainted with a lot of the pain of growing up trans in a time and place where there wasn't much visibility or support. My younger self had to survive so much rejection and erasure, and on the precipice of parenthood I realized how unfair and overwhelming that was. Yet I also feared that being so sad would somehow close me off to being able to invite in and support new life. As I was sharing this with a friend one evening, she went into her house and came back with a very small ivory box. Within it was an even smaller rosary. It wasn't a religious offering, so much as an offering of connection, to know that my younger self and my current self were being held. This prompted me to go home and create a conception altar with items that helped me feel connection—to community, to nature, to the big moments in my life, to the universe and to the possibility of conception. I began sitting at the altar on most days, sometimes alone and sometimes with my spouse, and she also began writing to my womb.

The morning after my LH peaked, my spouse and I did a small puja at the altar as we waited for the midwife to come perform my IUI. We anointed the gods and goddesses, the rosary, the shells, a jar of glitter a close friend had sent as an offering. We treated everything as holy. And then we sat. I breathed in and felt the breath stretch down into my womb, into the core of the earth, and out into the universe. For the first time in my life, I became aware of my ovary as it began to release the egg that would become one genetic half of my first child.

In the months that followed, my spouse and I continued to use the altar space to ground us and started to think about the rituals and traditions we wanted to carry forward in the family we were forming. Each time we sat, I felt a deep connection with the being growing in me. It all felt very natural and obvious, as if these links and these practices were lying dormant in me, in each of us, in our relationship, and that calling Sanchal in just awakened this whole rich tapestry of connections for our family.

It's now been a little over two years since losing Sanchal, and I find that they're still such a significant part of my spiritual practice. Part of this has been around learning to perform certain rites of passage for them as well as for my living child, because our family wouldn't be fully seen or honored if we were to seek these services from a priest, but it's also what takes shape as I continue to parent a child who lived so briefly in this dimension. We've spent time together in dreams and in visions. We've held each other and cried together. I've comforted them and offered them freedom to go and to return home when needed, and they've offered me forgiveness. In my second pregnancy, their blue-green energy swirled protectively around the frenetic and joyful orange-reds of my second child. Each time I visit the place where we released Sanchal's ashes, I feel them powerfully. In the ocean waves, in the wind-worn cliffs and towering evergreens, in the albatrosses and gulls diving on the horizon. I still feel them in my womb, which has been a portal to entirely other planes of existence.

Simon: Thank you for sharing this, Aakash. Hearing about your experience at your conception altar, rites of passage for Sanchal, and journeying together with both your partner and Sanchal makes me think about the dimensions of life that are available through spiritual practice.

I feel a certain sense of mourning that I didn't have my current spiritual practices when I was pregnant, and also when I was going through pregnancy loss. I think I would have given myself more room to be aware of and feel into the dimensions of my experience, and my children's. I did take prenatal yoga classes, and we had time in guided meditation with our babies. That was very special to me but was just a few minutes a few times a week. I was in a bit of a valley in my spiritual journey, I suppose. I do remember feeling an enormous sense of being part of the human lineage, that I am a drop in the river of life, but also that I was a link in the chain of human existence. It felt both overwhelmingly special and exciting and also like the most ordinary and quintessentially animal thing to do. That sense of connection to the past and future also extended to other forms of life on our planet, and to our place in the universe, which still sparks wonder and awe in me in a way that is a spiritual experience.

One of the milestones on my journey since then is work that I have done as part of understanding/healing after my hysterectomy.

What I thought of as an organ that I no longer had a use for and a cancer liability was also, as you said, "a portal to entirely other planes of existence." With the help of a dear friend, I have been able to honor and release my uterus and find another seat for the parts of my spiritual self that were disrupted.

Zillah: My mom always told me that there are no coincidences. She died a few months after my child's first birthday. Nearly every day I think that my child was here to replace the loss of my mom. Though no one can replace my mom, the emptiness of the loss of her is filled with the everyday busyness of my child. My mom always wanted to be a grandma, and though it was not how we all envisioned it going, she was able to be one. Nobody really knows how anything will go once a new person is born, no matter how much I planned prior to my baby's arrival. I am happy to have had my mom with me through the pregnancy and the first year. I do believe that some divine intervention was part of that, especially with how sick she was.

What does it mean to be a parent who exists outside of gender norms and expectations?

Aakash: I am in a monogamous, monoracial relationship with a femme-presenting cis woman, which means we are very quickly read as a cis, straight Indian couple. There is often an erasure and invisibility to our queerness, to my transness, and to our roles in creating our children. There are many difficult aspects to this, including finding spaces that can hold all of us—in our grief of having lost our first child, in our identities and roles as parents, and in our decision to parent our child(ren) without imposing a gender identity onto them from birth. However, it can also be a lot of fun to watch people's minds twist around as they try to understand us. It helps that we have a shared sense of humor about it. Soon after we brought our living child home from the hospital, a neighbor asked my spouse if she was breastfeeding. While my spouse did briefly induce lactation, I quickly answered to say, "I'm the one that gave birth." The neighbor seemed stunned before blurting out, "Well, see, it goes both ways!" Still don't know what she meant by that. Another very sweetly brought over some heavily gendered gifts for our baby, whom she decided was a boy, and included a onesie that said, "Just like Dad, but tiny." It was so wrong, but somehow also totally right. I'm curious to see how things will be as my child grows to be school-aged. I imagine them having a lot of clarity and pride in our family, which includes a dead older sibling, a gestational Appa and a nongenetically related Amma, plus a sperm donor whom they might choose to contact one day. Their chosen family is a small circle who refused to leave us alone after my first child was born and died, including our loving midwife. I hope being born into this family offers them freedom. I hope their freedom helps shape a freer future.

Zillah: It's taken me many years to self-identify as trans-genderqueer. I've always felt I couldn't claim any trans label because I was Assigned Female at Birth (AFAB) and I have not done anything to alter that (i.e., no hormone therapy or surgery). There are many reasons that I've chosen to remain in a socially female-presenting body since puberty. One reason was based on the social narrative of what trans "looks like," and my self-denying closeted feelings led me to believe that was not me. I was stuck in the lanes of "this" (transgender with medical changes) or "that" (not being transgender because of no physical changes) versus all-encompassing (being transgender without medical-based physical changes). Through my teen years and early adulthood, I stifled being genderqueer and presented as extravagantly overly female. To me, this was basically many forms of drag, playing being straight and cisgendered. I had fun with it at least! Punk-woman drag. Goth-woman drag. Hippie-woman drag. Indie-woman drag. A blend of many-women drags. I look back in hindsight and think of myself as beautiful in all these different forms of finding myself, but in the moment, I struggled to see my own beauty, as it was much like dressing up for theater to be adored as a false character. Later in life I dressed more masculine. I represented who I am outwardly as socially male-like. I finally felt like myself: a trans man who still appreciated drag. The word *genderqueer* was my first word I had to understand myself apart from my cis heterosexual friends, and like a favored middle birth name, I still hold on to it for safety and familiarity.

When I became pregnant, a lot of my physical body changed, and I slipped a bit in my own trans self-acceptance, while simultaneously loving my pregnant shape. Between the clothing changes and my postpartum body, I felt like I slid back into my twenties, dressing in femme drag most days. When I look in a mirror now, I see myself as physically closeted no matter how verbally loud I am about being out. I often feel like an impostor. In the last few years, mostly post-pregnancy, I've learned that it's possible to be a femme-presenting, transman, gestational parent. I didn't have to pick a singular lane.

Under this body suit and gender dysphoria is a feminist man. I don't, nor do I want to, don a beard. I don't want to take meds and change my voice. I want to grow my hair long and eventually have it be white/gray and wear my favorite drag of all: a crone faerie. I wish I could remove my chest, but a lot of other things must happen before I fulfill that. A big part is acceptance of the scars that will remind me largely that I wasn't assigned male at birth (AMAB). I wish I had a clear path like so many other trans-folx I read about or hear from in trans support groups, but I know I am not alone in that my path doubles back on itself many times and isn't linear. I have a lot of fear of retaliation from society. I was raised in America in the "don't tell" mindset. Now that I have finally come out, the nation is taking away trans rights more than before (including taking away what equal rights others have already fought to receive).

I alternate between she/her and they/them pronouns, influenced by anxiety about the potential reactions and possible consequences of being heard from unknown individuals within society. I also cringe when I hear she/her, especially from my extended family, but I do not request otherwise. I also get self-conscious about being treated differently or further alienated by my extended family, whom I already lead a different life from.

Furthermore, I am concerned that my own uncertainty about switching between she/her and they/them pronouns may create a situation where my family becomes unsure about how to address me. Although I have a good sense of understanding myself, I frequently feel lost; to borrow Octavio Paz's phrase, "I walk lost in my own center." I often feel like I am behind on coming out as trans-genderqueer, and therefore being a parent is just another added layer to my internal dialogue of "Am I doing this right?" The question asking what it means to be a parent outside of gender norms is heavily snowballed into what it means for me to accept myself outside of socially gendered expectations, being a parent or not.

J.F. Gutfreund

Body Count

The changes are slow at first, creeping. It's hard to know what's in my head. I can only compare this to very early pregnancy. The sensation is a little flutter, vague nausea, and the thought that everything you know is about to change. A feeling in the nervous system, a subtle change in the tides of the inner ocean. I distract myself from overthinking. Everything is heightened even though I am not adrenalized.

I am thirty-one and have delivered a couple hundred babies in the last three years; my feelings about being a midwife are complex. There is a sense of conditional belonging. I can be here only if I am useful. Only if I am smarter, faster, and more productive than most. Only if I never bring up the inconvenient truths that my trans body offers to stories about birth. This dynamic is something I have agreed to, being halfway present in every interaction. Looking back, I can see this is a practice that is familiar to my body—something I have always done and not had words for.

I withdraw the needle and wipe the injection site reflexively. There isn't any sensation as it sits in a pocket between the fat of my belly and the muscle wall. When you read about testosterone therapy on the internet, it says terrifying things. It says you will get diabetes. Your blood pressure will rise. Your hair will fall out. You will get fatter, aggressive, and have mood swings. As I prepare my forty-year-old body for another transformation, I worry about my liver, my blood pressure, about the hair on my head.

I lie awake on the beige Berber carpet of a cold double-wide outside of Santa Fe at 3 a.m., waiting for a baby to come. I have been up for the better part of two days, and I am desperately tired but cannot fall asleep. There is a vibration in my lower abdomen that I have never felt before. Twenty-five days into the fifth cycle of inseminations, I know I am no longer alone in this body. I don't have joy or fear, only wonder.

In September, the season change starts to become apparent. The cottonwoods have yellow tips before I notice the shift in temperature. Blood moves downward, even while I am still celebrating the warmth of the end of summer. The river by the house is filtering the silt from late rain. I dip into it carefully. I want the full desire of midsummer but feel hesitant.

After only a few months of gender-affirming hormone therapy, the story I have told about my body starts to unravel. I want to quickly weave everything back together. To recycle all the storylines into a new, logical narrative about who I am. But really, there's just raw material. It's tendon and collagen, heart and blood, celebration and loss. All the practiced vignettes of my performance suddenly feel so naked and curated. Each an attempt to respond to the defining question of my life: "Are you a boy or a girl?"

I arrive at the hospital with my young client who is struggling after thirty hours of labor at home and no baby to show for it. I rush to get her comfortable on an awkward hospital bed with thick, crispy sheets. "So you must be the father?" the nurse asks kindly as she enters the room to check us in. "No," I say, pausing a beat to consider if laughing will make the situation better or worse, "I'm the midwife." The response is a familiar withdrawal—she looks down and hurries out—a tiny would-be connection broken because there is no story to hold this interaction. The whispered notes of shame and embarrassment on someone's face that I quickly assume ownership of.

I have resisted the "wrong body" narrative. I wanted all my dimensions—a story in which I get to be everything I am without experiencing the repetitive heartbreak of being misunderstood by those both far away from and close to me.

To be a parent and not a mother, a midwife and not a woman—and even the less tangible building blocks of identity that have told me I can't be masculine and tender, assertive and nurturing. To live inside the stories of my experience without having them collapsed into a story that's been heard before.

I thought if I could get my mind right around all these contradictions I didn't need to change my body—there would be nothing wrong with me, nothing to "fix." My carefully crafted middle ground weighed heavily on the philosophy of "You get what you get and you don't get upset."

At thirty-six weeks pregnant, I attended a birth at a family home twenty minutes outside of town. I love these clients; we are warm and caring to one another, and they laugh easily at every prenatal. She is a labor and delivery nurse, nervous to be birthing at home and excited to be the first in two generations to approach it.

I am dragging. My legs swell insistently when I sit too long, when I stand too long—they are never satisfied with their position. The grandma is so kind and fusses over me, forcing me to lie down while I wait for labor to advance.

We have been pregnant simultaneously for months, her third and my first. So many similarities we groan and chuckle about, eating furiously at 3 a.m. on an overnight shift and trying not to vomit. The differences in our stories are there too—her pregnancy clothes fitting around the shape of her belly with form and function, the many times a day she is asked, "Is it a boy or a girl? Could it be twins?" versus the rarity of these questions from strangers to me.

As someone well versed in the social conversations of pregnancy, I notice people do not ask me much, and I do not offer. It is winter and I am covered up. The changes feel so catastrophic inside me that I can't imagine others do not notice, including those who I am offering care to in their pregnancies, but in fact many people I see regularly fail to notice I am pregnant. Somehow at thirty-six weeks I am still "coming out" as pregnant on a regular basis.

Feeling seeps in, spreading through the corners of my body. Waves of awareness begin to flood me. I didn't have the wrong body; I had no body at all. The rush of sensations is something I was not prepared for. It hurts with goodness; it shocks like truth. My body unfolds layers that have been tightly tucked away. Each layer makes physical a dimension, a new part of the form. It's a field of flowers right after the rain. It's the enchanting breakdown of leaves into dirt, it's the germinating seed bank that's invisible right below the surface.

Pregnancy is not dysphoric, but public life is. I refuse maternity clothes; the empire waist and capri pants aesthetic of maternity wear doesn't exactly hit the mark for a tall transmasc who usually fits easily into men's sizes and shapes. I wear my jeans unbuttoned under my oversized button-downs until my partner sews a panel into them. I look at my body in the shower; it is so different, and as strange as it ever has been. My body feels like an exploding rainforest—a TV time-lapse of exotic bright-orange efflorescence under a dark canopy. Rapid transformation is awe-inspiring and in sync with whatever it is my spirit knows about purpose and place, while life outside wears the same gray fog of misinterpretation that I am so used to. Not always injuring, but an endless map of missed locations that seem like they could have been shared with others, visible to me but not to them.

The baby is born quickly and is caught by her own mother, who brings her to her chest and cries with joyful relief. I sit adjacent to her legs, watching for the telltale signs of a good transition—gush of blood as the placenta separates, the grimace of another contraction after so many, and the lengthening of the umbilical cord telling me it is unattached from the inside. Instead she begins a trickling bleed, a continuous red rivulet forming under her.

I tighten internally and my body goes quiet in the familiar way that happens when I am about to react. My voice stays calm and my hands go through all the usual motions to pull up the medication that will try to coax the bleeding to stop: syringe, vial, alcohol swab, needle to thigh, injection. Blood comes in a thicker stream now and no placenta still. My hand follows the cord into the ridged balloon of her uterus, fingers formed in a scoop. I shear cotyledons of soft, slippery placenta off the sides; they shred into my hand. She shouts, "Keep going!" while I do this. I bring my hand out with another wave of crimson fluid.

I kneel in the back of an SUV with the seats flipped down, putting compression on her lower belly as we drive to the hospital, where she will stabilize and be reunited with her baby once again. It is only then that I see how ridiculous this is—me, only a few weeks less pregnant than she was earlier this evening. Hunched over, keeping her uterus clamped around a wound the size of a grapefruit, eager to spill out at the slightest relaxation. This is the last birth I attend before I give birth myself.

Only occasionally at first, I let my body show up in the room around me. I become less afraid of how much masc or femme I'm performing on any given day. I start to feel things that were previously locked under the shielding of automatic response. I look cashiers in the eye, and I start to smile when I'm pleased versus trying to please. I quit things that don't let me show up as a whole person.

The winter feels long. There is snowfall in March and April and even in May. On my due date, four inches of heavy, wet snow falls in front of the house. It melts off by evening, making all the pathways into mud ditches. I wear my winter boots and walk five miles every day to keep my blood pressure down and to make my mind quiet.

I go past forty-two weeks of pregnancy, and everyone is distraught about how to get this baby to come. I spend untold hours pumping and walking and taking concoctions that make me vomit in hopes of inducing labor at home. I have contractions all day, and every night they go away. My baby moves and grows and stays put. My midwife tells me, "I still don't really understand how you identify, but I know it takes deep feminine energy to give birth, and I need you to find that in yourself." I stop calling her for help.

It is shocking how good it feels to have a body. I am filled with longing. I suddenly feel as though I have never been touched—never received touch in the way I can feel it. My skin burns lightly; there is a tiny breathing forest on my outer layer, gulping in the carbon dioxide of my environment, sighing out oxygen that fills the air around me. It is both longing and satiating simultaneously, the closed-circuit reciprocity of embodiment.

Nursing is the thing I fear—not sure of how I will be able to bridge a relationship between my chest and any other body. I have not tried to do so for at least a decade or so. I have anxiety dreams where I am trying to get the baby latched onto my belly button or other places that don't make sense. My partner and I imagine a scenario in which we both nurse the baby and dream up ways how this precarious labor could be shared.

When they are here, it is not easy but not impossible. I stay up all night bringing them to my shiny, swollen chest. I coax them to try a little harder, open their tiny mouth into a slightly wider gape. I hold their soft feather-covered head in my hand as they nuzzle and root and then scream out, nuzzle, and root again. At last they latch on. There is a stabbing pain in my shoulder blade so intense I fall out of my chair. I slide onto the floor, keeping my baby held to my chest. They drink with deep relief.

At eight weeks, I go back to work, that is, go back to attending births. We haven't been separated up until then, not even for a few hours. They do not appreciate my sudden absence and go on a nursing strike. For the next month, every time I try to nurse them, they scream out like they are in pain. They gag at my chest, and struggle and arch back. I take to putting them to sleep before latching them on. I sing and hum and rock and rock and rock at the first signs of their hunger. Their resistance grows my commitment stronger. I feed them from my body, and we are reassured that this was meant for us. We are, after all, still mostly made of the same body for a little while longer.

I walk in a drenching spring rain that has caused hundreds of worms to crawl out of their holes, littering the road with their mucus-filled bodies. I wonder about their struggle—pushed from underground by the oversaturation of life-giving water that suddenly fills their bodies and makes it impossible to breathe. I see my own body, a delicate mauve sleeve, gasping from the doses of essential resources at toxic levels. Struggling to inch toward homeostasis while risking deadly collision with the forces of nature.

There's a way we are when we are not absent from our form; it's a body count, beating. The truth of my body seeps out into the air around me, having the effect that it might have, however drastic or unforgivable, however mundane and unnoticeable. Of course, there is softness too—the tickled recognition of my loved ones, as I emerge from places they might never have dreamed I was contained by. "You look gooood," breathes my trans beloved, staring into my face for a moment longer than usual.

There are walls I have adapted around—the ones holding me together and holding me back. I have wrapped around the hardness inside again and again. The tissue layers of protection form a criss-crossing pattern that can't be undone with a unidirectional approach. I wonder about the love I have received, with its unsaid story about what one must be to be loved.

At nearly forty-three weeks of pregnancy, I take myself to the hospital for an induction. The staff know me from transporting my patients to this very same labor and delivery unit. They are only a little self-satisfied seeing their local midwife come in for a medical intervention. I decline a gown and I keep all my clothes on. I wear my T-shirt to the dissatisfaction of the nurse. I take my pants off only when my water breaks. They are cordial with me as a patient—calling me "she" and "mom," inquiring about the details of my too-long pregnancy.

Once I start having contractions in earnest, I close my eyes and don't look. The immensity of the pain swells take me into a world where I am not self-conscious, not guarded, only clinging to the short moments of stillness in between, asking my body to open. I can feel my partner there; it's all that matters. I do not see when they swat her hand away as she reaches for our baby as they emerge. I do not see anyone. I feel every inch of my baby arrive into this world; I replay this spectacular feeling over and over again in the following months. They are placed on my belly, blue-tinted skin pearlescent with fluid, eyes closed, not ready to look just yet.

I start to get a flutter of excitement on injection day. It's a feeling of anticipation. I allow myself to imagine what might change and how much more I could feel. My voice cracks and I listen in my head as though this person is in the other room. I hear a resonance that sounds like me. There is a curiosity about myself that hasn't always been there; often I have not been curious at all. Some of the fractures are inching back together—integrating. I try to reach back to the child who wanted to know how to be these things all at once. I offer this to them—"Take it," I say, "it was always yours."

Lífthrasir Green

What It Was Like to Have an Abortion

What it was like to have an abortion:

I took the train downtown, which sounds like a great way to get pregnant, but in my story, it was a way to get un-pregnant.

I walked to a neutral-looking office tower, found the neutral name of the neutral clinic, and took a neutral elevator to a neutral hall. I entered the nondescript door and was greeted warmly by a radical-feeling receptionist, which would have felt normal in any other setting in my West Coast city, and I guess I should have expected people working at an abortion clinic would have a good vibe, but somehow her realness shocked me. I was having a very beige experience and somehow the full-color presence of the receptionist being there for my full self was jarring.

I got a clipboard with papers, filled out the papers, returned the papers. The papers included questions about my prior pregnancies (four), births (two), my pronouns (he/him), my surgeries (none yet), my medications (none yet). I had brought a craft project—a baby sweater I was knitting for a friend.

The waiting room had windows and a few other quietly and temporarily pregnant people. Magazines, television, a bowl of condoms. I worked on my project and hoped my act of baby-focused domesticity was not triggering to the other people in the room. It soothed me, to create in an act of love, when I was on this slow-moving assembly line of disassembly.

My name was called. I followed the person into the room. I was cheery, because I'm cheery by default. I was grateful for the kindness of the person, and said so. I was grateful they do the work they do, and said so. They were kind to me while they asked their questions, and I didn't feel like they thought I was a shitty person for choosing one family shape over another family shape, for missing out on the sweet little life that could be a big whole life. I felt like they were taking good appropriate care of me while the sand of reality was *huff huff* shifting just a little, like the ground might be solid but might just slip away into the stars.

I was given a gown and time to put it on, knock at the door, awkward "Come on in," ultrasound, confirmation of pregnancy (fuck fuck fuck fuck fuck). I don't know really what happened then, probably a gentle yet efficient exiting and entering of the room I sat still in. Still, and still pregnant. Officially pregnant. Officially pre-abortion. I had not yet been offered the abortion I had gone there for, based on a home pregnancy test, which maybe could have been not real, but the official pregnancy test and the ultrasound were real. So I was really pregnant, in the year that and with the person who for so long had been part of my Life Plan, but things had gone wrong and it was all sideways and fucked up and I was still pregnant.

I don't know why, but I wanted them to know I was one of them: a feminist, an activist, a smart person. In hindsight, I think I was having a very important transition, an unwelcome rite of passage, and I wanted to be seen and held. And the fucked-up part is that there were people in my life available to see and hold me! The two people who knew I was there were really in it for me with all their hearts, but I didn't talk to them about my feelings, just about how to pay for it. I also had dear close friends I should have told, but couldn't, because I didn't want to make it real. Instead, I created a void between us.

The trans-friendly doctor prescribed me the medication and talked gently with me about what to expect and under which conditions to contact their office or go directly to an emergency room. I went home and took the medication and bled and cramped and bled and bled and uncontrollably lost my insides and my blood and my heart and my embryo and the vastness of space wildly all over my clothes and the tile floor. I raged like a hunted and caught beast. I was beastly, bestial, bloody and powerful and lost and sad, and somehow taking the steps on the path that was the right path. That was an act of faith, faith that my loved ones knew what was right for me even though I was too disoriented to make the decision myself.

And how her shadow, not really a shadow but more of a twinkle, is still with me. Two years younger than my youngest. What would she love? What would irritate her? How tight would her curls be? I imagine her as a firecracker; I picture her being a little too bossy for her friends—figuring out how to be a leader. I guess she is whatever I imagine her to be, which is so much easier than the real thing.

For that, I am grateful. For the real thing, and also for my precious child who never was to be, who is whatever she might have been, and also who was spared all that I was not able to be.

My heart aches for her, these many years later. She would have been amazing, but I would not have been. I did the best thing I could do for our family. Oh, my sweet little one, let's the two of us just be exactly what we are, because what else are we going to be?

Zillah Rose

The Home I Made for You

To my Grandma M. and Mom, who both told me to write more

I found out I was pregnant with Catkin when I went to the ER with my mom for an unrelated health issue. Being assigned female at birth, they took my urine to test for pregnancy before I could agree to a CAT scan. When the doctor came back and said he couldn't do a scan because I was pregnant, my first response was, "Shut your mouth." Ha. Then I said, "I don't believe you." The doctor did a quantitative blood test to check my HCG levels (human chorionic gonadotropin, a hormone produced by the placenta during pregnancy), and they were quite high. I was convinced at the time that I had cancer, and I worried about that until the vaginal ultrasound. This was my initial reaction, as multiple tests over the years had suggested that I would never be able to conceive my own children, and that if I wanted a child that was genetically related to me, I would need to seek out a surrogate service. One of the main reasons I struggled with conceiving and having a live birth is that I have Trisomy X. This means that I have forty-seven rather than forty-six X chromosomes. I want to mention this to normalize genetic chromosome mutations, especially for those of us who are genderqueer. Trisomy X causes a high probability for early menopause; some people go through this in their early twenties. I started perimenopause when I was thirty-five and rarely had a cycle. Due to my age, having Trisomy X, and having had a couple miscarriages in my early adult years, I was told by doctors that I would have a high-risk pregnancy. I felt like I held my breath the whole time I was pregnant with Catkin, in fear of losing another fetus.

During the nearly nine months of my pregnancy, my family and I experienced several significant life challenges. I also happened to be pregnant during the first year of the COVID-19 pandemic. The main challenge was that my mom had metastatic breast cancer. We were lucky that she was gifted the time of my pregnancy and the first year of her only grandchild's life. A silver lining of the pandemic was that I was able to isolate myself with my parents and share a lot of precious time together both during my pregnancy and after Catkin's birth. When Catkin was a newborn, my mom would soothe them by simultaneously whispering, "I love you, I love you, I love you," along with the standard "Shhhhh." When I was young, my mom always made sure to tell us often how much she loved us, even when she was hungry and exhausted from running a household and raising two babies. My mom, exhausted and then with cancer, was there all hours of the night telling both Catkin and I how much she loved us and lulling my newborn back to sleep so that I could sleep too. My mom mentioned time and time again how much it meant to her to have known her grandchild before she died.

I wanted to start my story about my mother, because she is as much a part of this story as Catkin and me.

Growing up, my mom supported and validated my choices to express myself however I wanted, even when she didn't understand my constantly changing assertions that "*This is who I am.*" When I asked to be called my chosen name instead of my birth name, she said, "I didn't know of the name you needed, and the name we gave you was the best one we could give at the time, but I am happy you know your true name, and I will call you that from now on." She rarely slipped up, and she always corrected herself. She offered many times to support me in changing my name legally, which I opted not to do. I still alternate between using they/them and she/her pronouns from time to time, but my mom said she would use whichever pronouns I wanted. She was the type of person who always had my back even when I annoyed her, and when I needed her, she let me come to her, or she would find a way to come to me. She was that way in her words as well.

Since it was the first year of the pandemic and people were unsure of how the virus spread, no one out in the community attempted to push unwanted attention on my growing belly. Despite all the tragedy associated with the global crisis, it wound up supporting me and my desire for time to nest and fold within myself and share special time with my mom.

I gave birth to my Catkin at a birthing center outside of the hospital. I had a doula, a few midwives, and my mom there with me. My mom did the honor of cutting the umbilical cord and bonding with my child alongside me. Prior to birth, my doula helped prepare some ground rules in case something went wrong and I had to give birth at the hospital. I feel like the stars aligned to have the doula I did. Though she was newer to queer terminology, she was dedicated to learning about me, my needs, my pronouns, and my parent pronouns. She respected my choice to go by "Dama" rather than "Mama" or "Mother" or "Mom." She promised to post my needs above the birthing bed and to be a strong advocate for my needs and boundaries as a gestational parent. I am grateful that the birth was successful at the birthing center and that they respected me by asking for my preferred pronouns on my first visit. They even crossed off my name assigned at birth and put my chosen name at the top of my charts!

While pregnant, I chose a parent pronoun that would best represent myself as a genderqueer parent. I wanted a name that was unique to me and that if my child yelled out the word at a Pride event, multiple other parents wouldn't answer. Looking at the English language and baby babble sounds, I thought about how babies say "Dada" and "Mama" and pushed them together to make the name Dama. I hoped that I would also be called Dada rather than Mama until my kiddo could put the two together. For a couple months, my babbling toddler called me Daddy, and I was totally fine with it. I found this endearing. As the world began to reopen following the first two years of the pandemic and there was more influence from the cisnormative community, there were a few months when my baby stopped calling me Daddy and started calling me Mama, as that's what everyone outside of our home called me. This made my skin crawl with gender dysphoria. I had a therapist who helped me unload that anxiety with reminders that this name would pass and that soon my baby would call me Dama. Sure enough, they did and still do. Now that they are a toddler, they will openly laugh in the faces of others who call me Mama instead of Dama and tell them that they are silly and wrong. I wish I could do the same without any repercussions and laugh at distant family who have a deaf ear to my wishes. Though I love the word "Mom" in reference to my mom, it was never to be my name. My mom supported that and corrected anyone she heard call me the wrong parent pronoun. I love the name "Mom" so much, but I also detest it so much.

Coming to terms with my postpartum body has been hard as well. That magical bubble of mental safety that I was in popped!

My body is not my body anymore. I have slightly bigger breasts than before, and they're more noticeable now. I feel like I will not be as much of an attractive genderqueer trans person in this body that feels so specifically and socially female-gendered. On medical charts for my kid, I am "Mother" and "Mom." I am called these names even though I protest and write calm, collected emails to my kid's pediatrician. I tell people in person that they can call me "parent" or "guardian," or if my parent pronoun name is too challenging, they can call me by my name. I try to be forgiving, but I still get frustrated and return to those icky gender dysphoria vibes I felt when my baby repeated the word "Mama." I know this is something that will show up time and again, and already it exhausts me.

I wanted to be pregnant so much. It was the only time I may have truly loved all my body as a larger-bodied person, as a person born with a vagina, as a person with more than one X chromosome. It was also the only time I liked having breasts, as I thought they would feed my child. I felt like I kept them around for that purpose only. When they didn't produce milk and didn't support the baby, I was quite annoyed that I had kept them around all these years! Though in hindsight, due to having to reach out to my community for breast milk donations, my child and I now have two awesome families who donated their breast milk and who have helped me build a loving and safe community: a chosen family. During the pregnancy, I loved all parts of me, even though to the outside world I was seen as "a woman who is pregnant and will become a mom." When I looked in the mirror, I saw myself as a gift for Catkin to grow in, just as my mom was the gift for me to grow in.

I was gifted with the ability to know myself mentally and emotionally as a person before I became a person who is also a parent. I worked hard on holding boundaries and having others ask for consent. The pandemic gave me lots of opportunity to prioritize the safety of myself, my child, and my mom, even when others were annoyed with all the N95 masks, COVID tests, and quarantines. I have no regrets about my firm boundaries around COVID-19 precautions, even though it caused turmoil with other family members. My mom's last months alive and her dying were all that mattered to the wellness of my dad, my child, and I. Spending the remaining time my mom had left while not making things worse with COVID taught me how strong I can be and gave me confidence to be true to my decisions as I figure out how to be a Dama, on my own, now that my own mom is no longer beside me and here to advocate for me and can no longer guide me as a mentor. I feel like the loss of my mom, upholding values that showed up surrounding the COVID-19 pandemic, and being a solo Dama have all taught me that I can get through the hardest of days. I believe that those same hardships can also be what support me when I am dead-named, called the wrong parent pronoun, and figuring out how to teach my toddler to use inclusive language in a society that does not support my being a Dama.

Following my own trauma and having lived in crisis mode for a good part of my life, I grew up seeking acceptance from other people to feel validated and whole. Though I did seek acceptance from my mom the most, and her view matters the most to me to this very day, I now must seek that same level of validation fully within myself. I often feel alone and isolated from other biological family members. I do worry about my child mostly having only myself and their grandfather as consistent bio-family, but I also want to teach Catkin how to pave new empowering roads without traveling within intergenerational trauma and seeking validation through that brokenness. I also want to teach my child the value of creating a fierce bond with friends as a chosen family. That said, I am very grateful that my dad is here and part of our daily life even when we are incessantly reminded of the heaviness of losing my mom—a compassionate and vivacious pack member.

Having my own child has been a new journey, and my life before now feels like chapters of a previous life. I feel the same way about the death of my mom. Though I'm not young, I felt like I was still my mom's child, holding her hand when I needed it. Now that she is gone, I offer my child my hand and do my best to support this person with as much generosity and compassion as my mom gave me. Having grown up feeling genderqueer and in fear of being rejected by my cis peers, and now being an adult who often feels like an imposter in most groups, whether that is with cis parents or queer/trans parents, I still hope that I can be someone my child can turn to in life, whatever their gender identity may be. I hope I can pass along to my own Catkin the same acceptance and kindness that my parents showed to me. I hope that my child growing up with a genderqueer trans Dama teaches them how to be who they want to be, even when the odds don't look good.

I hope we rise and thrive in defiance despite all the people who use laws and religion as weapons to diminish our existence.

My and Catkin's birth journey has purpose and meaning.

Jacoby Ballard

Trans Body Magic

My child is a magical being. She is free. She is authentically, unapologetically, and uniquely herself, both because of who she is and because of gender-expansive and queer parenting. It is a gift to be granted the honor of being her parent, and I am ever grateful that I chose to carry and give birth.

During my germination, my partner and I moved from the queer haven of western Massachusetts to the Mormon-founded metropolis of Salt Lake City for my partner's tenure-track job. I was skeptical that I would find adequate providers, and I held low expectations, familiar with the track record with queer folks of the LDS church, which until recently provided conversion clinics for "same-sex attraction." Unbeknownst to me prior to landing in Utah, Salt Lake City has a thriving community of birth workers, and within the breadth of this community were indeed some queer and trans-affirming providers.

As a queer herbalist and plant lover, I named my experience *germination*, a process that describes a seed growing into a plant, a magical process that sends plant life from the dirt into the sunlight, fed by the nutrients in the soil and moisture. Queer folks have a culture of creating new words to describe our lived experience, and this extends into queer conception, pregnancy, and family building. We often use unique words for our family-making process, our body parts, our parental titles. Renaming my experience as *germination* felt more inclusive and embracing of all of who I am, and less gendered than the word *pregnancy*.

To my surprise, my embodied experience of germination was fascination, as someone who works in the field of embodiment. I remained curious throughout the changes of forty weeks and three days of being pregnant: the nausea, the uncharacteristic attachment to macaroni and cheese and aversion to anything green, the movement of the baby in my body, how my partner could feel the baby's kicks when I spooned her, the incredible growth of a new organ through pregnancy. I learned about amniotic fluid tasting to the baby like the food I was eating, introducing a child to their cultural foods. I learned about how much blood my heart was pumping through my body and the baby's body. I felt the top of my rectus abdominus muscle ache as my belly expanded, and I became aware of the inside of the right side of my rib cage, which my child burrowed into.

My partner delved into researching birth and translating the materials into queer narratives and stories that were not just centering pregnant cisgender women and narratives about husbands and cisgender male partners that varied from presence to a lack of involvement. My partner was also the first line of contact with people we considered bringing onto our birth team, providing a screen for any transphobia we might have encountered from providers who were meeting me for the first time.

The birth team we assembled consisted of a midwife who, twenty years prior, had been a women's studies major at Goddard and Prescott Colleges, a midwife's assistant who is queer identified, and a queer doula with a transman partner. I took a birth education class from an instructor with a huge heart, humility, and determination that allowed her to greet her two trans masculine pregnant students with grace and a warm embrace. I had a queer acupuncturist, a parent herself of a child now in his twenties. Through my experience, I learned that in the state of Utah, queer and trans-affirming birth is possible!

I was not interested in learning about the baby's sex before they arrived and asked that not to be revealed during the ultrasound. I knew that would provide fodder for all kinds of projections about who the child was, their interests, innate gifts they embodied, colors of blankets we were given, clothes. In fact, anytime my partner or I experienced one another projecting any kind of hope or possibility onto our child, such as "What kind of artist will this child be?" or "I can't wait to shoot hoops with our kid," we were in a practice of offering a counter-narrative: "... or maybe we have a kid who is afraid of balls or wouldn't set foot on a basketball court." This practice helped us be collectively aware of expectations of any kind and created space for our child to be exactly who they are.

Because of my partner's screening, I largely didn't have to interact with providers who weren't a good fit for our queer family, or for me as a trans masculine pregnant person. There were a couple of mishaps with two providers, a prenatal yoga teacher and a prenatal acupuncturist; I am grateful that these were exceptions to the norm, and it feels worthwhile to write about here as a learning experience for fellow seahorse parents and providers alike.

In a prenatal yoga class that welcomed both the birthing parent and the partner, we had asked that the teacher not indicate in any kind of obvious way which of us was carrying the child. We knew that because of our gender presentations in a setting like this, my partner would read as "woman" (she identifies as non-binary), and it would therefore be assumed that she was the pregnant one between us. This was a way to protect me from any invasive questions that could be asked by fellow students, allowing me just to be a participant in a yoga class and not a gender educator off the clock. However, when we walked into class, the teacher came right up to me and asked in a loud voice, "So how far along are you?!" thus making it obvious that I was germinating, not my partner. There were three couples present, one pair being two queer women, and I did not feel endangered; however, this moment broke trust with me and I did not return to this prenatal yoga teacher's class.

The other moment was with a queer cisgender acupuncturist. She had known that I did not want to learn about the baby's sex, including from a Chinese pulse reading. However, she did just that at the start of one of my sessions and told me the baby was female. I went on with the session but told my doula about it, who had recommended the acupuncturist and had a relationship with her. I was not interested in shaming the provider, but I did want her to be aware of how her conduct did not align with my request. The acupuncturist immediately reached out to me and apologized, regretful of this breach. She offered me a refund on the session, and I continued to see her through the end of my germination, having received a reasonable repair.

Because I was new to Salt Lake, I didn't have much interaction with "strangers"; rather than dealing with the common comments from strangers that cisgender women who are pregnant receive, I was invisible. This saved me from unwanted conversations, but it also denied me public recognition of what I was undergoing, an experience of invisibility common to pregnant transmen. On a work trip in New York City at around five months pregnant, I was riding a subway packed with people, being tossed around by the turns of the train, and I feared falling and injuring my child. I read the familiar sign that advises riders to offer their seat to elders and pregnant people. I was faced with the choice to out myself (or be presumed to be a woman) and receive a seat or to remain standing and invisible and endure the discomfort and fear for the duration of the ride. I chose the latter, one form of safety over another.

Trans-Embodied Birth

I wanted to have a home birth as a protection from transphobia: I knew that in a hospital, I couldn't control who would enter my room or the discussions that would take place at the nurse's station, whereas in my own home, my partner and I could set the culture. We were prepared for a possible hospital transfer, complete with my partner's thorough flyer that articulated our parental titles and roles. (I was carrying our child, and my partner had induced lactation.) I am grateful that we got to stay at home.

As a trans yogi, giving birth was the most embodied experience I have ever had. I trusted my contractions, and when I felt the urge to push, I pushed. It wasn't consciously effortful; the effort was just in allowing what was happening to happen; my body just knew what to do. My labor began on a snowy January morning and lasted six hours, and I pushed for maybe twenty minutes. My communication regarding anything outside of myself was limited and curt, whether regarding the doula's pressure on my hips or the birth assistant taking my temperature. I was clearer on my needs and preferences than I had ever been; I was completely and fully in my experience, an internal focus familiar in meditative states.

My doula at one point demanded that I look in her eyes: "You can do this, Jacoby," she reminded me firmly. As contractions became more intense, I dug my nails into my partner's shoulders, leaving red marks visible in photos. At one point, the midwife came and looked in my eyes and apparently used few words; I just understood her psychic instructions. Then she said aloud, "Jacoby, standing is a perfectly fine position for giving birth. If you want to birth in a squat, you need to sit right now." I sat on the squatting stool, and my midwife invited me to touch the baby's head. I was giving birth! I may have smiled. The next contraction pushed out Gigi's head as I groaned, and then her shoulders and body tumbled out in a big squishy blob, right into my partner's embrace.

As soon as our baby was born, I came back into the world. Sounds and smells returned. I was attuned to the breath of my baby as my partner and I held him between our chests. He cried loudly and shot a fountain of pee into the air, announcing himself and anointing us as his parents. Shortly thereafter, we were cuddled in bed, our baby latched to my partner's chest, the two of us fed from the nourishing food in our refrigerator. After a few hours, the birth team left, and I remember thinking, "Oh no, what do we do now? They trusted us with this precious life?" I had so much to learn about parenting, and so much internal knowing about love and showing up to just tap into.

The most gender dysphoric experience I had was after birth: wearing pads in my boxer briefs for weeks. No one had told me about this part of the process! The pain in my crotch, the incessant bleeding, and the bulky pads I wore (soaked with herbal medicine for quick healing) provided an experience that ranged from awkward to enraging. However, since healing from birth, bleeding monthly is no longer dysphoric: It reminds me I have the power to create life, and that I did just that.

Prenatal Yoga

I am a yoga teacher, and I have taught yoga in studios and at many different sites over twenty-five years of teaching: a recovery center, a cancer hospital, an organization supporting unhoused people, queer bars, social justice organization offices, art galleries.

During my own germination, I only attended two prenatal yoga classes. One experience is detailed above, and in the other experience the teacher was great, but I felt out of place and not necessarily welcome or understood by the pregnant women in the class. I continued practicing yoga, making adjustments in general classes but not necessarily preparing my body for birth through my practice.

I didn't come out to my students as pregnant until my thirty-ninth week and was generally assumed to just be a guy with a sizable belly. I was new to Salt Lake City and didn't have long-standing relationships with my students, so they didn't necessarily know that my body is usually different.

The yoga studio I worked at prior to giving birth had pledged to find a substitute teacher for my classes and then allow me to return to teaching once my body had healed from birth. However, just before I gave birth, they changed the titles of all my classes and gave them to other teachers. When I inquired about this, they terminated my contract and sent a cease and desist letter. Although it is illegal to fire someone who is pregnant, most yoga teachers are independent contractors for a studio and therefore not protected by workers' rights, workers' compensation, or antidiscrimination laws. As I know from a previous experience of transphobic employment discrimination in New York City, it is difficult to prove discrimination even in a state that protects people from discrimination on the basis of gender identity, which Utah does not. Thus, just before giving birth as a trans masculine yoga teacher, I lost my work with no protection and no recourse.

After giving birth, I was asked by a prenatal yoga teacher training program to write an article about my experience, with some recommendations for prenatal yoga teachers. This endeavor led to being invited to lead LGBT-inclusion workshops in several yoga teacher trainings. For over a year, I cultivated a wonderful relationship with one such training that emphasized reproductive justice, and then attended the training as a student. After the first session, I provided feedback, which the instructor appreciated. Recognizing the labor of that feedback, she offered to refund my payment for the program, stating that the feedback and suggestions were ample compensation. That recognition and generosity was so healing for me, for my gender experience to be seen as an asset rather than a threat. My trans siblings, this is the standard of treatment we should expect; cisgender colleagues, I invite you to consider the concrete, tangible ways you recognize the labor of trans people you work with.

For the last four years, I have offered Queer- and Trans-Centered Prenatal Yoga as an online program, accessible to students all over the world. I welcome and include cisgender and straight pregnant folks, while prioritizing the experiences and conversations most pertinent to queer and trans folks. It is a pleasure to hold space for queer family making, to make an offering that I would have benefited from so much myself. As my colleague angel Kyodo williams says, "If you don't see something in a space, that's because it's your offering to make," an instruction to release resentment and accept the invitation to create what doesn't already exist. Attendees of my prenatal classes have a variety of gender presentations and parenting arrangements and build relationships with each other across time and space. My class is offered to help mitigate the discomforts of pregnancy, to make space for the spiritual inquiries surrounding birth, and to serve as a training ground for the birth experience.

Experiments in Gender-Expansive Parenting

My co-parent and I have been committed to gender-expansive parenting since my germination, aware of the damage the gender binary can cause to so many of us, and interested in what happens if we don't parent in a way that conforms to the expectations of the gender binary.

Our child was assigned male at birth, and in the beginning, we used he/him pronouns (rather than gender-neutral pronouns), mostly because we live in Utah and I, as a trans parent, didn't want to be fielding the pronoun discussion at every school drop-off or playground encounter. We have told Gigi, in child-appropriate language, how our family was made and who played what role. She has known that she is a seahorse child and that I am a seahorse papa since she could grasp narratives and stories; she knows that what is required to make a baby is an egg, sperm, and a uterus but that those elements can be present in a variety of different bodies. We taught her about her anatomy and that of others and have maintained since the very beginning that people of any gender can have any variety of genitals.

Choices for children remain so gendered, from toys to clothes to extracurricular activities. We knew the world would throw everything considered "masculine" at our male-assigned child, and so we skewed toward the feminine, trying to ultimately achieve a balance. We use gender-neutral words such as *parents*, *grandparents*, and *kids*, and we have avoided providing a narrative about the gender binary. Gigi has always had many trans, genderqueer, and non-binary people in her life with a variety of non-gendered titles, such as *guncle*. When Gigi was very young, we dressed her in dresses and pants, really anything cute, and largely shopped in the "girls" aisle at the consignment shop. (The clothes are just cuter!) We have honored her interest in construction vehicles, and also decorated them with sparkles.

What we found, after Gigi was two years old, was that she had a genuine preference for all things shiny, sparkly, and colorful. I once bought her a pretty basic REI long underwear top for forest school when she was four years old, and she scoffed at it, saying, "Too plain!" From early in her life, because of her clothing and hair that has never been cut, Gigi was read as a girl on the playground. After a Day of Trans Visibility rally at the state capitol when Gigi was four, she told us she is trans and asked to use they/them pronouns; six months later, she said she is a girl and uses both "he" and "she" words. When she began identifying as a girl, we didn't know if it was a mirror of the world assuming that she is a girl because of her hair and dress, or because that is her authentic identity. We imagine this may change, and we are here for the ride of her own self-discovery.

Along the way, I have told Gigi about my own experience of being trans. When I tell her about the discrimination I have faced due to transphobia, from being fired for being trans to being called her mom, she snuggles into me or gives me a kiss. I am clear that I am not looking for her to take care of me in that moment but that I want to share with her, through my lived experience, that the world can misunderstand us or be hostile toward us as trans people. So far, I haven't told her about laws here in the state of Utah and nationally that criminalize our use of the bathroom and prevent her from participating in sports divided by the gender binary. I want to protect her from that fear for as long as I can, while ensuring her safety and supporting her interests. I want to give her time to root into who she is, to have that deep knowing before the world casts doubt or asks for proof. In the extracurricular activities she takes part in, my co-parent has written up an incredible one-sheet explanation about who Gigi is and how teachers and instructors can protect her and treat her well; so far, her swimming, climbing, and dance instructors have been enthusiastic about protecting and supporting her.

It is quite a joy to share a trans identity with my child, even as we have different gender presentations in the world. I never would have anticipated that fellowship as I became a seahorse papa. My child schools me in gender sometimes: If I use a pronoun for someone I don't know, she corrects me, telling me, "You don't know they use a 'he' word, Papa." She scoffs when we enter a binary toilet and celebrates gender-neutral toilets. She knows that families and love can look so many different ways and that no way is better than another.

My child and our relationship give me hope for the better world I've been working for my entire adult life: She is free from the gender binary, expects to be treated with kindness and honesty, and greets others with curiosity and generosity. My experience giving birth connected me more deeply to my body's power and capacity, and I feel more deeply rooted in my trans body, heart, and mind than before germination. I feel more trans than ever, a further becoming of myself through my perinatal experience and parenting.

Conversation: Community

Did you know other people of your gender who had been pregnant? Did you talk to them? What did they have to say?

Amber Hickey: Yes! Through a great pregnancy group with JB Brown that I did during my first pregnancy, I met some other nonbinary pregnant and postpartum folx. The whole experience was very affirming and made me feel more empowered in my own birthing and postpartum process. It felt like I wasn't in it alone, because many of us were struggling with intersecting challenges. I wish I had queer pregnant community like that this time. I think it's also more difficult this time because I am around more people generally. Last time, it was still peak pandemic and my bubble was small, so I did not have to do quite as much emotional labor to address cases of misgendering. People often assume I am cis until I tell them I am nonbinary, and that has always been even more pronounced when I'm pregnant. I feel like I'm starting all over this time, having to be really clear with people. I know that I am not alone in that experience, and it continues to be a challenge.

Kara Johnson Martone: I am the first queer person I knew to get pregnant. I found a lot of community, and resources, through social media and our doula (who was queer). I am always excited and proud to make connections with other parents who identify as queer and trans and currently run a support group for queer-identified parents.

Aakash Kishore: I'm getting caught up on the words "your gender," which . . . no? But yes, I did know a couple other trans/nonbinary folks. How we navigated pregnancy was very different, because the world experiences us very differently. For instance, one friend who had been on T longer than I had before stopping to have zir baby decided zir safest route based on where ze was living would be to present as female for the duration of being pregnant. Having rather robust chest and facial hair, that would not have been possible for me, and working a government job at the time meant I couldn't change my insurance marker to female without changing my gender marker across the board. One thing ze said did really resonate, though. We were talking about the loneliness of an invisible pregnancy, and ze spoke about connection to a lineage of other trans, nonbinary, and gender-expansive folks, some who had walked a portion of this path before and some who would walk a portion in the future. Perhaps we might each feel alone in our own moment, but we are a part of something much bigger.

Simon Knaphus: Before I was pregnant, I was able to find one other FTM who had a baby. I emailed him and he sent me a really thoughtful and encouraging email. When I was still pregnant with my first, I met a lovely trans couple who had a toddler, and who then had another baby shortly after my first was born. We had a lot more in common than just being trans people who had babies, and they were some of my favorite people to spend time with. We talked a bit about pregnancy and birth, but because we had little ones, we talked more about parenting than pregnancy.

What would a world with real reproductive choice look like to you?

Tom: The first thing that came to mind was reproductive choice experts that represented an array of experiences and backgrounds to support. Reproductive choice would mean reproductive justice that includes systems and laws that are more inclusive.... As I write this, the list goes on, but realizing the work ahead is so long. Glad for this conversation—feels like a little step closer.

Simon: I love dreaming really big about this. I imagine a world in which reproductive choices aren't made for us by economic factors—we all have access to the material resources to shape our families however we want. No more, "I want to have kids, but I can't afford to." To me this also means universal health care and excellent free childcare, and the freedom to choose whether to access childcare or not. I like to expand this to community resources too: that we can expect our cultures and communities to affirm, honor, and celebrate our choices. If we choose to have kids, they will be enthusiastically welcomed. Real reproductive choice would mean that we wouldn't have to worry that our children would experience discrimination, war, environmental devastation, or other human-made systemic harms. I also love to imagine radical biological choice: that anyone who wants to be a gestational parent can have that experience, and that anyone who doesn't want to doesn't have to, and that our choices might change over time. Same goes for feeding babies and for being a genetic contributor/collaborator who is not the gestational parent. In a world with reproductive choice, many family shapes would flourish—solo parents, co-parents of all stripes, monogamous couple-led families, poly families, people who choose to have families without children, families where nonparents raise children who they love because they want to, so many options, and all where kids are never an unwanted burden or an unrealized longing. All people get to choose if and when they parent, with whom, and in a supportive environment without threats of unnecessary hardship or social pressure either way.

Kara: To me, this means that all medical professionals would have information about queer families and their options for childbirth. When I think about choice, I realize that in that initial meeting with my ob-gyn we were not given any options. There was one option, and that was the path we went down. I wish that we had at minimum been given resources and information about queer birth workers and nontraditional methods of conception and childbirth. Unfortunately, I don't think this is something that most doctors currently have.

Aakash: I agree with everything that's been said. I would also add that with real reproductive choice, folks of color, and Black folks in particular, would not experience disproportionate rates of pregnancy complications, fetal loss, and death. This would probably mean reshaping so much of how health care is delivered and reimbursed, where everything from medical education to reimbursement algorithms wouldn't be based on young, able, thin, cis white women.

g k somers

Stardust and Magic

I felt you waiting there, long before you had a chance to spark and grow. I could hear you like a whisper; gentle, following me everywhere. I thought about you every day, until one day, you started becoming; stardust into small seed, and then you grew to become you.

I remember the first time I saw and felt your heartbeat—so quick, like the wings of a hummingbird. I remember observing your tiny fetus on the monitor, some eight weeks after you were conceived. Thumpthumpthumpthumpthump.

The first time I felt you move, I lay in the clawfoot tub of my apartment in the West End of Vancouver. I felt your foot swoop against my right side. I would become intimately familiar with that sensation as you grew and stretched your legs often ... your feet always dancing.

You were head down from the get-go. Just waiting. Ready for the world.

Growing up, I never wanted to be a mother, even though I was always good with kids. This is to say that the dream of becoming a gestational parent wasn't always with me, but neither did it pop up suddenly overnight.

The shape of becoming a birthing parent became clearer as I discovered language for my gender and new forms for my body ...

I was eighteen when I first heard the word *genderqueer* and twenty-three when I began my medical transition. It was sometime around the latter when a friendly acquaintance, Addie, asked if he could interview me about being trans for an article he was writing in journalism school. It was over tea and discussion in his kitchen that I named out loud that one day I might carry a child, and that being trans didn't prohibit the possibility, it enabled it.

From the other side of the room, Addie's partner, Dev, shouted, "You should use Addie's sperm! You two would make beautiful babies!" and this was the start of that seed.

There were a handful of times in my late twenties when I thought I was ready to start trying, and each time, something held me back.

Each time, I'd ask myself a new set of questions, and at the core was, *Am I really ready for this? Do I really want this?* And finally, I was, and I knew that I did.

It was June 2020, and we were still in a sort of lockdown from the COVID pandemic. My roommate/chosen brother, Caz, and I had just moved to the West End after both spending many years in East Van. Summer had brought us more openness to connection, but everyone was still cautious. I bought a paddleboard and spent most days paddling the inlet.

I had gone away camping with a couple of friends during the July long weekend, and the seed sparked again.

My friend, while we were camping, asked if I still planned on having a kid. For the first time since I thought it up into being, I wasn't sure. The uncertainty didn't last, though, because within a week or two, I reached back out to Addie to ask if he was still open to the possibility of being a sperm donor. I met up with him and Dev in a park near their home.

I pulled out paperwork for us to look over and asked the kinds of questions that would allow us to get clear on what this agreement would be. He didn't want to be a father, and I didn't want a co-parent. He filled out all the paperwork related to genealogy and readily went to the fertility clinic to get his sperm assessed.

In September 2020, I was on my way from Kamloops to Penticton when I realized I had my last dose of T before my vial would empty. I pulled over to the side of the road, gave myself the shot, then tucked the empty glass vial away for safekeeping. I wrote a spell, tucked it next to the vial, and got back on the road.

Less than one month later, my menstrual cycle returned (the day after my birthday!), and with that, I began tracking.

Addie was living out of town at the time, so we discussed the possibility of my first DIY at-home insemination happening in December, if timing lined up with when he was planning on visiting.

It did.

The morning I called you in, I walked down by the water. It was gray and a light rain fell. I laid down prayers and watched as a heron took flight. I saw Addie walking along the seawall.

We hugged and went to my place, just up the hill. I handed Addie a sterilized cup to make the deposit while I made tea.

I set candles and lights, and waited, sipping my tea.

Addie returned from the bathroom, holding a cup with the thick, viscous liquid that would help conjure you. We hugged and said goodbye, and then I went to my room.

Two days in a row we did this process. One of your *tías* came by after round one. She laid her witchy hand on my womb and helped with the conjuring. *Did I mention that you were made of magic?*

I got the keys to the new apartment, a place that felt like home from the moment we stepped foot inside. There was a working fireplace, a clawfoot tub, and enough room to grow. On the night of the winter solstice (the night after the second insemination), we went to the apartment, lit a fire, and I called you in, wishing you into being with all my might.

Community collaboration

Dreaming family, lineage and place relations

I gave what felt like two hard pushes—my hand inside me, cradling your head

You have hair, I said aloud.

The first push

You crowned

The second push

Your head came out

The third push somehow took less effort

As your shoulders slid forth and the rest of you came effortlessly out . . .

At least, that's how I remember it now.

03h47

As you were placed upon my chest, I remember looking down at you and saying

Welcome, Echo Dae.

You were/are, perfect.

Later, your Uncle Chris would remark, "Yeah, you were remarkably lucid!" Or was it in the moment? I can't quite remember. All of time seems to have collapsed in on itself.

I was four months pregnant when Zee and I met, and I fell in love quickly and wholly. Evenings were spent paddling on the water after work, taking long walks, and having deep talks. *It's not every day a pregnant trans person falls in love during a pandemic.* After one month of knowing each other, I let my feelings be known, and to my luck they were returned. This is the person who would become your *amaapa*; your *apa*.

Months five through nine were bliss. Spring bloomed into summer, and I was happier than I've ever been, feeling fully aligned and exactly where I was meant to be in my life. As you grew, I grew, and our family grew. Zee and I adventured, taking trips to the island and staying in my dear friend's old VW overlooking the ocean. I whispered love murmurings in that van as Zee lay behind me with their arms wrapped around us and hands resting on my belly.

You and me, we would return to that VW time and time again in the first couple years of your life.

Your due date coincided with the day that Zee was to start their PhD. That night, we went out for dinner in the neighbourhood, then walked to the beach nearby. We sat by the water and waited. I knew you weren't coming; I always knew you would arrive a week later.

I still didn't know your name. I thought I did, but it wasn't quite right.

Your name came to me in a dream.

The next evening, I sat on the lounge next to the window at Zee's and wrote your name for them to see. Echo Dae.

That's it.

On the day leading up to the night you were born, Zee accompanied me to the hospital for what would be my final ultrasound. In and out real quick, the technician told me that everything looked good.

That night, we let go of knowing when you would arrive, only for you to make your way into this world just hours later.

0001—a stabbing pain more intense than anything I'd ever felt, and then fluid was everywhere.

I rolled off the side of Zee's bed and ran to the washroom in time for the rest of the amniotic fluid to leak into the toilet. Zee brought me my phone, and I called the midwife. She said not to panic, that it could take several hours for the baby to be ready, and that I should try to go back to sleep, given that the baby likely wouldn't arrive until the morning. She said to call back when my contractions were five minutes apart.

I did not feel like sleeping.

I let Uncle Chris know, and Zee called Caz to let them know we were going to be heading back to the apartment. I called my mom and told her not to worry (she wanted to know when I went into labour) and that we'd call her in the morning.

The timer ticks, another contraction hits. How long has it been? Not that long ...

Zee and I get in the shower, thinking that I've got time to rinse off before getting in a cab to go home for the birth. Another contraction hits. We get out of the shower, Zee calls a cab, and fifteen minutes later we're home.

I start puking and shitting myself. This is the part that no one seems to talk about. The contractions are the most painful things I've ever experienced. Caz reminds me that my body is probably in shock from the pain, and, somehow, this calms me. My contractions are already two minutes apart, and when I realize this, a part of me panics. We call Uncle Chris; we call the midwife; both are on their way.

I lay on the couch, and each contraction brings more pain than I've ever felt. The moments between contractions, I melt into whatever surface I'm lying on.

Words and people are a blur, and I somehow make my way to the floor.

Then I am standing and swaying, Caz behind me, my arms on Zee's shoulders, until the next contraction hits and I drop to the floor. Caz catches me and lets me down gently. I'm crying and, suddenly, Zee's arms are around me.

The midwife arrives at some point, but I'm not sure when, sometime when I am still on the couch. I remember her voice coaxing me to the floor ... Chris guiding me.

I only ever wanted to bring you into this world with the help of people who wanted you here. I wanted you to know that you would be loved by every person I brought into our lives. You would never feel a lack of love. You were born of dream magic, stardust, and love.

I'm sitting between Chris's legs now. Caz is somewhere to my left, and Zee is to my right. The midwife is standing somewhere nearby. I know this won't go on much longer, as I've already decided that there's no way we're going through contractions all night long, and there's no way that pushing you out will hurt more than this. So I ask you if you're ready. Echo Dae, are you ready? I can't do this without you.

I hear your yes, and I push.

Interview with Amari Ayomide

I sat down with Amari Ayomide on a beautiful spring day to talk about their experience of pregnancy. Amari works with Queer the Land and is parent to a fifteen-year-old. They had just returned from a week of learning in Cuba about Afro-Cuban land stewardship. We met again later by video. This interview is a combination of those conversations, edited for clarity and length.

Simon Knaphus: It's so good to meet you! Thanks for sharing your story! Let's jump in. What was your experience of gender and sexuality when you were pregnant?

Amari Ayomide: There was just a kind of expansiveness. You're carrying this human life inside of you, and then you see this human life come from you in so many ways, and you're just like, "Who's to say what body, what gender, gives you this?"

Pregnancy allowed room for an expansiveness that brought more questions than anything, but it also pushed me to stand my ground a little bit about who I was. I either was gonna let those people decide who I was, or I was gonna decide for myself. And even though I wasn't sure, I just remember myself always fighting back from those narratives.

That, coupled with the expansiveness of being in my body, and whatever experience I was having, I literally was just a body carrying another body. It kind of gave room and gave way for that.

I experienced the violence of transphobia and queerphobia being pregnant. I was very mainline lesbian at the time, and then I "wasn't" anymore. And then, the violence of going through these shifts and motions where that was very much a talking point for people who were like, "You were saying you're a lesbian but you're pregnant," and literally being asked by my dad, "Oh, I thought you were a lesbian." It forced me to be like, "*Am* I gay? And what is that? And what does that mean?" And then kind of pushing myself up with a more openly queer identity because I was like, "I'm gonna prove to you how fucking gay I am." Ummm, that was a fun time of my life.

I had longer hair at the time, and I fully cut all my hair off and had a mohawk. That was my first time doing anything like that, so I was very proud of myself for that. I always look back and reflect on nineteen, after my baby, being the time I really came into my queerness because of how much it was questioned while I was pregnant.

I was understanding and learning that I could confuse people, that was fun for me, because I had spent so much of my time confused and very dissociated from who I was and what I could be. I think that actually was a huge guiding force in my androgyny and my mix-matching. It was my way of reclaiming that kind of gross toxic confusion and harm that was perpetuated to me as a pregnant femme-presenting person who was *fighting for their life already* in Black queerness, living in whiteness.

Simon: Do you want to talk about your son's birth?

Amari: It was this very surreal experience, because even while I was pregnant, I didn't really feel connected to being pregnant. I think, with my PTSD and neurodivergence, and then also my transness, I was experiencing a lot of dysphoria. I was also experiencing a lot of cognitive dissociation from myself. I think for me it's important to acknowledge that it wasn't *not* a joyful experience, but it wasn't this ethereal experience of like, "I'm a parent now. I've had a baby." It was very much in its own right, its own existential experience: that I just had a baby. "Oh, my God! I carried you for nine months for real, this wasn't a joke. This wasn't a dream."

I had this very light-skinned, crinkly baby in my arms, and I just was like, "Wow, [he] looks so like me, but so unlike me." It's kind of a disconnection, but also a connection to the ethereal experience. Very surreal, like, "Oh shit, this is happening," but also just like, "Oh, this is happening. What am I gonna do now? How do I go from here? How do I take care? I know the next step is breastfeeding." I couldn't do it. It didn't feel comfortable to me, and nobody helped. I wasn't given the experience of being told about breast pumping and things like that, so I didn't have that experience of the baby feeding naturally from me, and I think that caused another disconnection. I had postpartum depression almost immediately.

Holding this baby, having this baby in my arms and being in this setting with no real connection to community or to self or to anything, was very ethereal, in a beautiful way and also not.

Thinking about it, it's so important to me to acknowledge that I had this experience, and it was also intercepted and tied to so many different things that I was also experiencing: my very, very, very wild and clear disconnection to womanhood. I don't know what a woman feels like. I know how to play the part, but whatever identity of womanhood that I expected to feel or expected to understand more, once I had the baby, I still had that disconnection and it just kind of furthered that for me. I think once time elapsed, it connected for me and I was like, "Oh, I'm not a woman." But at the time it kind of just hurt me.

I think that we put a very wild expectation on parents, just period, but the cis hetero parenting experience was not there, and I think I kind of expected this mommy gene, or even a parent feeling. Even before I had a baby, I was like, "I'm the dad, I know I am," and not because I even identify as male or even really masculine, but just the gestures, what I knew to be a dad: distant, disconnected, you know, kind of like *the boss*, the one that steps into the relationship and is like, "No, Mom said no." I thought, "That's definitely me," because I didn't feel this motherly or parent-y connection to my child.

I think also what made me cry was that I did not feel connected the way I thought I was going to. I did not feel connected at all. I was just like, "I'm holding this baby that came from me but does not feel like it's mine." So it took me a while to be like, "I'm a parent."

He was separated from me for eleven years. Now I'm more in his life. I think that also was very scary for me moving forward, because I just never felt that connection as a parent. I didn't know what I was doing. I felt like a person who had a baby and there was a lot of expectation to show up and to be whatever, and I think that I held that against me for a long time. I've had to really create a new relationship with parenting now, especially just because of the trauma and experiences that we've had, and even then, looking back I always felt guilty for that. But looking back and reflecting on it now, and looking at my parenting now, I recognize that you have to create your own relationship with that, especially when you're not given *a single fucking tool* to be able to. So yeah, there's a lot of disconnection. And I used to feel really sad about that. But, in hindsight, I'm like, "What did I expect, you know, like what?" There shouldn't have been anything more expected from me than what I was able to give.

Simon: What are some of the other tools or resources or community supports that you could have had that would have set you up for a transition to parenthood? If things had been ideal, what would it have looked like?

Amari: Community is not just the friends and the other families. It's also the practitioners, the level of care, the doctors. Having a gender or sexuality coach or doula would have been so helpful and supportive. I was very queer, but I had framed myself in this box of lesbianism, and then I was having a baby, and people were disgusted. And then, having a birth doula who is actually there to care for my needs in particular, to the feeding and things like that.

I've never really been disappointed that I couldn't breastfeed my child, but I'm disappointed that I didn't get the care that I needed around it. For months I walked around with hard breasts. In my brain I was like, "These look great because they look like breasts I've never seen or had on my body, and I have been dying to fit into this form of femininity." Right? But they hurt, they feel bad, and nobody is really sitting down to tell me what I can do, how I could have been feeding my baby from my body. Actually, I could have been pumping. I could have been pumping and giving my baby breast milk.

You know something, I was kind of processing this a couple weeks or even days ago. I'm not thinking about having another kid. But I'm like, "Oh, this is what it is to feel like there's a possibility to bring more life into your life because you have a support system." I think, this time around, if I did it, I would absolutely be equipped from every possible angle. If I could avoid it, you would not catch me going into hospitals. I would have all at-home care up until birth. The one thing I would settle on is going in for giving birth, getting an epidural, and being there for a few days, and then getting the fuck out.

I would have all that care. Even at this big age of my transness, I would have a gender doula. I would have a support that could be with me as my body changed, because I also understand now that uncontrollable things are fucking happening to me, that no matter how big and bad and trans, it will make me question my identity, and so I would definitely have that support. I would also have some type of navigator that could help me navigate social service systems. If I could have a harm reduction specialist, if I could have a personal support person, if I could have an eating disorder support person, or a dietician that was actually about supporting me and the child I'm growing—if I could, I would have all of those things and have it all well broken down to me, as if this is my very first time. You need all aspects of care. Right? And you deserve to have every facet of your life taken care of when you're literally carrying another human child in you.

Simon: Absolutely. Yeah. The picture that you paint of this supportive network of specialists and navigators and people who are tending to you. I love that. Do you want to say more about your relationship with consent and your body during pregnancy?

Amari: Understanding the ownership of my body was really important, because for the first time I was experiencing a level of consent that I hadn't before, even if it wasn't a full level of consent. People asked before touching my belly, and even though people only noticed my needs because I was carrying, my needs actually did matter. It did matter if I ate three times a day. It does matter if I drink water. It does matter what I'm consuming and not consuming. I think those were really important factors of being pregnant that I subliminally carried.

The ways that I looked for care and nurturing were much different post-pregnancy than they were pre-pregnancy, because I was just looking for a basic connection pre-pregnancy, and I would take anything I could get. I think post-pregnancy, because of that experience, I really did learn that there's a different kind of connection and a different level of care that people will give you or you can receive. It is much deeper than surface level.

Simon: What was your experience of community when you were pregnant?

Amari: When I was pregnant, there was a very strong sense of community, and people wanted to protect me adjacent to carrying a person inside of me. I think that's important to note, because that, in and of itself, creates a dialect of community that we don't generally tend to understand or have access to. If we could hold on to that a little bit more, *as if everybody was carrying a something inside of them that was important to people*, I think that would be so beneficial to community.

I was feeling a lot of disconnect once the time came to have Baby. It was like, "Oh, y'all actually didn't really care about me, you cared about this infant." It was like disconnecting the parent from the child in a way that both don't matter, and like having that interconnected relationship doesn't matter.

Did they ever think that parenting is a reflection of how the parent cares for themself and how they have access to care for themself? We have these systems of CPS, and we have these carceral systems of parenting because we disconnect the parent's access to the way that they're able to parent the child. Not being in relationship with the parent as a human and just as a vessel is a very important characteristic of my experience.

I mostly grew up around white people. A lot of my friends at the time were white. A lot of my community at the time was white, and so that also plays a huge role into how I was cared for, and that community disconnection of like, "We care about the baby, and you're holding the baby so we'll care about you right now, but after that we're only going to care about the baby," whereas maybe in a different community, I would have been cared for a little bit differently.

My son's biological father is Lakota. I had spent some time on the reservation a little bit with him, and it was a nightmare. I was not welcomed into the community, because he had spread a lot of misinformation about me. There's a lot of anti-Blackness that I faced there. So again, I did not get to experience community in the ways that I think I could have during my pregnancy. I think that it really taught me a lot. It furthered some of that distance I felt, but also taught me a lot about what I actually deserve, or what I was actually capable of receiving at the time.

Simon: It sounds like it gave you a taste of something to look for, both in what you didn't receive and also that what care you did receive could exist in a different way.

Amari: Yeah, absolutely. And I do remember just being pregnant, soaking up all the affection that I was getting, it was so much different than what I was receiving at the time, but also just still feeling very disconnected from it in a way—but obviously a lot of that care wasn't about me.

But yeah, that sense of community. That makes me think about that community that I had when I was pregnant. The white people that were like, "Oh, look at you beating all the odds, being a Black parent."

They didn't say that, but they didn't have to, because the expectation shifted immediately once my child was born.

The way that I'm seeing life function now really just deepens the understanding of that need for community. The understanding that you deserve to have during that time, during that very special sacred time of holding a baby in your body for nine months. You will never have that time with that child again. That is the most special and sacred time that actually should be all about you, especially as a trans person, and especially as a queer person, and especially as a multiply marginalized person, and especially as a person of color. That time should fully be about you and supporting you a hundred percent, so that you have a basis and a premise going into this of what that is for yourself, because parenting is actually less about the child and more about discovering who you are as a human being, and who you want to be, because, if not, this child will show you.

[Our earlier conversation] brought up all of these feelings, this desperation and need for community that I didn't have, and made me feel that disconnect of what it was like when I was pregnant and not having that, but now I'm experiencing life and experiencing community, and I can also see the beauty that was missing. The real beauty of the community was just getting to have the experience of a baseline of understanding who I am as a person, as a parent, and how I'm going to be treated, and how that completely shaped how I chose to move as a parent, because that's such a sacred time. I hope that this story can invite folks to understand how important their autonomy is during pregnancy, and that it *is* about the child, and in order for it to be about the child, it has to be about you first, and this is your time to figure that out. Yes, you have plenty of time, but this is your sacred time, while this baby is in your body, to figure that out, and do not let anyone take that from you.

Simon: Absolutely, and the importance of community is something for people outside of the pregnant person to hear. It shouldn't be pressure on the pregnant person to all of a sudden build community. It should be that when someone in your circle is pregnant, that's when you really show up and be part of this sacred process that you're privileged to be a party to, in a way.

Amari: Yes, yes. Are we thinking about the experience like that? Instead of being like, "You're a person who holds this child who has this duty, who is supposed to do this thing." Yes, yes, that's exactly it.

It is also extending the hand to community to understand, too, that this is a sacred time for this person and your place is actually to live up to deserving that space that's not given to you, just as much as it's not given to the parent. The parent also has to do their work during that time. So I appreciate that. That's exactly what I'm trying to say, 'cause we're not just telling these stories so that we can feel better about ourselves, we're also telling these stories so that you can hear what we need from you. When I say I was lacking community, I'm not actually just blaming a system. I'm telling individuals to get up off their ass and do something too, because it's not just the system. You can be more supportive by listening to what our needs are, and [we need] to be given the opportunity to have external chances in our favor, to be able to figure out who we are as people and who we want to be, while our body is literally transforming in front of us.

It is so invisibilizing, to be trans and a parent. You can't understand my experience as a Black person, but you can understand my experience as a trans parent and how invisibilizing it is. Queer parenting was actually normalized in the 1990s, and gay men started to centralize their life around the cis/het white male experience, and so these gay white men that beat the odds of the epidemic of AIDS, if they had it or not, then started building queer families. They actually normalized queer families in a way that is helpful to a lot of us, and also isn't, because of racism and all that shit.

Simon: It opened one door. And when we had our babies, both of us, it was during the gayby boom.

Amari: Yeah, yeah, exactly. We were having them naturally. I don't know how you had yours, but yes, I did get pregnant by a man, and I did have sex with that man, and that's another aspect of it too.

There was this normalization, from the '90s on, into when we started having children. It was like, "There's queer people being parents, but there's still not normalization of trans people being parents, and you have to fit into cis-heteronormativity. You have to put your shit on." You know what I mean, like, "God forbid! I'm a 'femme-bodied' person who has a child now, but I identify as trans, but I don't have top surgery. Sorry I'm not running around, and my boobs are already cut off, and I already have the surgery, and I'm pregnant now." Then you kind of normalize it. But that's still not normalizing trans pregnancy. It's normalizing a still further cis/het form of trans pregnancy, which is difficult to say, because then you get into the like, "Well, I'm still ..." That's very true, but you need to understand the complexity of where you're at right now. You are visibly trans in a way that people understand: the surgery. You've had the surgery. So you're trans now. And now you're emulating that experience and creating or living your life doing what you should be doing. But you're also perpetuating an experience that doesn't exist for a lot of us as trans people, if you're not talking about it.

Simon: Yeah, and we're all under a microscope to prove our identities, to prove how we are as parents, to prove that we are male enough, or queer enough, or trans enough, or whatever. And that comes from so many places, that comes from the straight world, but also trans people, it comes from other parents, it comes from queer community.

Amari: Yeah, it does. It comes from all of those things, and I think the key part is talking about it. Please live your trans-est, queerest, whatever that means to you. Please normalize that for us, but also please talk about the experiences that are missing and find a way to encompass them in that. Even if you're just like, "I'm grateful to be a trans parent, but I also recognize that many trans parents aren't gonna look like me. They're not gonna have the income I do. They're not gonna have the two-parent household. This is not about normalizing cis/het parenting in a trans way. It's about normalizing the trans experience in a multiplicitous way, while still honoring the experiences of people that don't get to have that."

I'm never gonna be able to go back and add what I have [now] to that experience. I think that is what hurts. It breaks my heart now. I never get to go back in time and say to myself, "It's okay, you. It's okay, you're trans, you're queer, and you're evolving. And you're making this possible for other people in the future." I have to live by that. So yeah, I think about that very often. I see trans parents, but they're not me.

So I think it's really great also that you're writing this, but also encompassing everybody. The multiplicity of people's experiences.

Simon: Thank you. I want it to be for all of us. And there's so many people who I know exist who can't contribute for many reasons. I feel like each one of us who shares, and the stories that we share, create a ripple effect. And I love that.

Amari: Somebody is gonna find their story in here. Somebody is gonna find their story. One thing that I've learned is that actually, my story does exist, and that I can be proud of my unique story, and I'm grateful that many people didn't experience what I did, but also, there is a story like mine out there, and there's somebody who has experienced that. I hope that if somebody reads this it's like, "Yeah, that's *woah*. I went through that same thing."

Simon: Absolutely! Or even if somebody says, "I see your openness to yourself and to your own story. And then I can be open to myself, my own story, even if it's a completely radically different one." To be like, "Okay, there's room for me here."

Amari: Yeah, yeah, I agree. Yeah, thank you for that perspective. Because I came back [to the US] believing that our biggest failure in creating community and creating liberation here in the States is that we don't embrace the norm. We actually have to embrace the norm for what it is, so that we can figure out how to transform outside of that norm.

We have to accept that we live in a carceral system, we live in a transphobic system, we live in an anti-Black system, we live in an anti-Indigenous system, because that helps us accept it within ourselves, and then we can mobilize to figure out how to do different. Otherwise, we're just like, "This sucks and we hate it!" And we spend so much time and energy just fighting that system with no understanding of that system and how it works, because we don't embrace it, and you can embrace it without holding on to the idea that it's real.

Now I want to figure out how to change beyond it. Maybe somebody sees this as their story. But also, maybe sees this as their ability to live their story, no matter what it is, no matter what your story is.

Felix Aster

This story, like a star, like a black hole that warps that collapses all, a flicker, a chance, bursts forth at the moment of birth and shoots outward in ten thousand directions.

Who am I writing this story to? When we three try to talk, signals cross and glitch. Sometimes we can't sit together without someone shouting or storming off. Sometimes we scatter like pool balls to our rooms, leaving the center empty. Sometimes we are a quiet sweet tangle.

In the cocoon of ketamine, in the depths of the darkest year since the birth, in a chair in a clinic high over the Salish Sea, I chanted the names of the triad of us until we became a loop, and the loop became one entity again, as I hadn't felt since early newborn days, when we were all naked and twined up in the bed skin to skin to skin.

Before that, postpartum, I lost my mind and my anchor. My worst fears—a looming figure, being shut behind a door, a loud threat from one parent to another—lay coiled in me like a black snake. I lashed out in the endless nights and bright days. The kid, only three, called me the mean one. I scared my partner. The ache and sadness—the gap between what we need and what we have, as Rod Ferguson said at a talk one night during that dark chapter—coiled into a knot under my left shoulder that ached in tandem with my heart. Each new stage of the baby's growth awakened another child in me, one that had needed what we were now giving the kid: touch, space, safety, delight.

That time we came to call the nightmare. One my own demons unleashed, starting a few days after the birth high. They pushed inside my chest and constricted it and battered the inside of my skull. I got to know them eventually, those protectors of bereft and angry children, to separate them one by one as they crowded my chest and neck and abdomen. In therapy, with guides, I learned to sidle up to them where they were stuck behind a locked door or alone in the sand. But before I did, I, in demon guise, lashed out and loomed and threatened my partner and, in so doing, scared my child.

I'm trying now to mend that rift. To understand it, first: the harm I caused my partner, our child, and the kin that shepherded us through the trans perinatal. I guess the truest thing to do is to write the story to each of us and to us three, and a bit to the larger circle of queer family.

Kiddo, I remember when you were not even a mote, but rather a chance.

I got you for a cheap bottle of wine on Sixth Street, on a foggy San Francisco night.

Tío D, he wasn't your *tío* yet because you weren't born, said, *Sure, come over, bring a bottle of wine.* He joked: *I guess we don't have to worry about the condoms.* We drank the wine, mostly he did, but I sipped a bit, for camaraderie and old times. We sprawled out under his sloping ceiling, the foggy night through the skylight. We kissed and tussled. Your Ba was driving in the Mojave somewhere. I called him on the way to David's and afterward, from where I lay in his little room in the boatyard building next to the Oakland harbor. Tío D said, *Light a candle for luck.* That luck was you.

Some of this is so intense I can't even talk about myself in the first person, so I'm using "you." I don't want the "you" that is me dissociating to get mixed up with you, my lover who I am addressing, but it's a mess and I can't tell who I'm talking to some of the time.

Lover, when I talked about having a kid, I had no idea:

Birth is a portal. The ring of fire, just before the head crowns. The endless dark before. Alone in a back room, only not alone, the baby is there too. The one we called the hyena, pushing and twisting and fighting to be free of you, the body that makes a warm wet home.

(When the kid and I talk about his birth these days, he says, *Could you hear me?* No, but I could feel you. *You could feel me kicking and pushing from the inside.* He grins at this—the scrappy wrestler he is, and was even back then.)

Alone, even if others are around, you can't really sense them, or, if you can, you can't reach them.

Torn open as you are.

The birth tears you open and the demons come out.

The midwives bragged to their text group, forty-eight-hour labor, twelve-pound baby. The baby posterior for most of that time, his spine pressed on my lumbar spine, stabbing ice pick, coccyx broke and then dislocated, the only time I could sleep at all in the last twenty-four hours was while leaning against my lover, standing upright, but then the pain got too intense and I pushed him away, snapped at him about how the candle was too bright, and told him to go sleep in the truck. The residue and shock is still there in the ache when the sacrum and the ilium scrape and catch on the left side.

Lover, I know you wanted to talk about all this then and tried to get me to talk or at least write about it. In the days after the birth, I did this, and what I wrote about was shock. It was bright noon. I was on hands and knees on the white flowered sheets. The midwives had me reach down and feel the head between my legs, it seemed superfluous since I had felt every hair and dimple on that head splitting me open like a melon. I see why they did it, to feel that moment of transition from inside to outside, from little hyena, sensed but not seen or heard, to little human, all mouth and shut eyes and soft downy hair on my chest. One midwife said the pushing would be the most painful, but when the head passed through my cervix I felt the excruciating coccyx pain vanish, replaced by a heavy fullness, like being fisted real good. The midwife had said that the next passage, through the birth canal, should be a gentle opening, with me holding back so as not to tear. Instead she was all quick orders—at me to breathe and to push, leg up, foot on the bed, and other brusque instructions. Her hands were inside me, stretching even impossibly more, dislodging the shoulders stuck wide inside me. Then: a surging flood, routing down and spilling across the bed, the baby's body slipping out all at once. Lover, you caught him and tried to hold him. You saw I was still in some other dimension. The midwife shouted to give the baby to me, I was trying to turn from all fours, I reached for the little fish and he slipped from our hands. The baby was a blue-white ghost on the bloody chucks, floppy as a fish, not breathing, all too human, but unworldly. I was so sorrowful, and also at a distance from him, this strange still doll. An image of the midwife bent, breathing into him, but maybe then he was already on my chest. I remember my certainty he would never cry, the endless expanse of that feeling, then she gives him two more puffs of oxygen and strips the cord blood into his heart, his skin turns pink on his face and his abdomen, though his hands are still so white. Then the midwife strips her two fingers hard down the edge of his spine and he gives a grating cry, to my loudest sweetest relief.

The demons attack your lover.

In demon guise, I blamed you, lover, for how alone I felt, how sore, how desperate for sleep and touch and comfort. In this dark cloud I demanded your care but could not let it in, your care or your needs. I shattered into parts that hurt and that pleaded and didn't remember what they had agreed or heard about what you needed.

Lover, I blamed you for not being in that birthing room the whole time, for not being able to get across to the midwives, who didn't believe me, how bad it was. I forgot, after we talked about it, that when they left me alone back there too long, you told them how much pain I was in, and they didn't listen. I forgot, until I read back in my journal from a few weeks after the birth, that we talked then about that long night. You told me and I remembered how you had told the midwives how much pain I was in, how they had said no one could be hurting that much and not be screaming. Later they said they didn't realize it was back labor, said they should have listened to me and to you about the molten stab inside my tailbone that never eased between contractions. But I didn't keep hold of this shared narrative we had created, and some part of me kept blaming you for abandoning me, even though you were right there.

The demons attack your dear ones.

The friends who come stay in the darkest fourth trimester chapter, dress the baby in the coolest onesies, and bounce him around the house so you can sleep. The others who cook rich decadent foods and make a family feeling. Those chosen family who see and fill a need with grace and shower the baby with attention while you, the one who birthed, and your partner are peeling up decades of linoleum and scraping lead paint off the walls on your days off from full-time jobs.

What I did in this state I can't remember. Or rather, my memory shattered into bright shards and some fell away into the void and some (most) were dislocated from any sense of timeline or narrative.

With undiagnosed tailbone fracture and dislocation, I couldn't sit without pain for six months, which a cis male doctor brushed off, saying, *Pain is part of birth.*

Terrified at the numb gloom I could not see through, the anxieties of gestational diabetes, lack of breast milk, lead in the soil, and store-bought formula flooded me and obliterated my sense of personhood. I expected everyone to see these anxieties as rational and do what I demanded. I lashed out, I behaved irrationally. I pleaded and then demanded—touch, sex, sleep—then retreated angrily and shut myself away when none of those things made me okay. I saw myself through a dark filter, saw my father in me like a black snake that wielded my arms and posture and voice, and my mother always numb and disavowing her feelings. I sank into a nightmare, became a nightmare, wielded a nightmare without meaning to, although intention matters little in the harm, in the rupture.

Lover, though I couldn't take it in for a long time, you told me: It was like at every stage the baby got to, you reexperienced all the pain of what you didn't get when you were that age, and you expected me or your friends to give that to you now, were mad at me and at them for not giving that to you, even though no one could give you that except yourself.

My parents put me in the crib from birth. I kept him in the bed with me. The kid, that is; my lover slept separately, so as to be able to sleep at all. And I saw the necessity of that and also was deeply lonely and touch starved on the nights I slept alone.

What I wish I could tell myself, the one who went off T eight years ago to make a child:

For me, being pregnant was okay. Yeah, I had bad nausea, back pain, borderline gestational diabetes, and was acutely uncomfortable from weeks thirty-six to forty-two as the kid grew and grew and had no intention of leaving. Yes, I felt alternately invisible and hypervisible as I envied cis women their sexy maternity wear and representation. But I felt held enough by the few trans masculine people I met before and while pregnant, by radical queer midwives, by straight women friends who, once they got over their shock that my beer belly held a fetus, connected over our shared embodiment and the strangeness and power of growing a child.

The biggest revelation, though, was progesterone, the miracle hormone on which I floated, as on a gentle sea. This second transition washed away my chronic anxiety and reversed my testosterone-induced hair thinning. Despite physical and social discomfort, I felt okay, more myself, fascinated by what my body could do and hopeful for a big move to a new city and job.

The birth began a rupture that tore those dreams asunder. Over years, trying to collect and mend the fragments with trauma workers, I came to see that postpartum plunged me into an anxiety-fueled psychosis. In that state, I did things that harmed my dearest ones and that left me flayed and bereft. We had moved, for work, to a new place with no net of medical or mental health care and not enough close family to hold us as I spiraled.

What is trans about this story, and what is just my own particular inheritance of intergenerational trauma flavored by white settler culture? Estranged from my parents because of childhood rejection, I found, in my twenties, anarchist outsider communities where trauma amplified in street protests and self-exile from mainstream communities. Traumatized in medical and mental health settings and dislocated from my support networks by a move away when the kid was four weeks old, I crashed and raged and felt utterly alone. I didn't fit at mommy meetups and didn't feel welcome at postpartum yoga. With a shitty doctor, I stayed off T for too long and waited almost three years to start mood stabilizers. Would those have been enough to keep me from shattering? Possibly, partially, who can say?

Over seven years, piece by piece, I resembled some sense of myself in the world, and I connected to people and earth beings through the crucible of the pandemic and my own and my lover's post-viral illness, held, however imperfectly and thus humanly, by queer family, dharma teachers, and trauma workers.

In the depths of postpartum psychosis, I couldn't imagine feeling belonging and delight in the world. I couldn't imagine a world or support system that could hold me up. Now I can see a haphazard one—that I have to pay for, that I could patch together because I lived in an urban center, that I could access weekly because of stellar group health insurance, that people on other insurance can't necessarily access, that is more clinical than I would like. This safety net includes therapists and body workers and acupuncturists, and also Buddhist teachers and sangha members who I contact over text threads and video streams and archived recordings of retreats. Piecemeal, I am cultivating a practice of stopping and deep looking, so I can see the joy when it's in front of me and feel into the suffering with an open heart.

As for so much in this neofascist late-capitalist system, it shouldn't be this hard to birth and raise a kid. Being trans, even with white and class privilege, can compound intergenerational trauma and makes it harder to access the imperfect social and medical support that is available to parents in the US. Outside the mainstream, trans and queer communities need to do the exhausting, connective work of making support systems for ourselves.

Maybe this story is a scatter of fragments, like clicks a bat sends out into the black night to find its food and find its way. *I invite my lover to talk through the draft, he says it wasn't like that, don't you remember? I tried to talk to you about this so many times, and you couldn't or wouldn't.* On the couch together, he tells me again, wary I will snap or lash out. This time, I can breathe a bigger space to hear him. How he felt anguished when I sent him out of the birth room. How the story I made up after, that he had abandoned me, made a trap he couldn't find his way through. These are some echoes coming back. Each one that hits my heart cracks it open a little, and then I can feel and hear and see a little outside of me, and feel a glimmer immersed and tumbling in the stream of life.

The kid sleeps with one of us almost every night, maybe making up for the baby nights when he slept alone in the crib, maybe just wanting that mammalian sweetness. He sleeps deep and hard, even when I'm hypervigilant or spinning out. We rarely sleep together, my lover and me, but sometimes we all three squeeze in my bed for a while, in a sweet tangle where the world is quiet and still.

Simone Kolysh

My body is a mother's body. It is not a young body with smooth lines from the thighs to the small of the back. Mine is a body of valleys, soft and reminiscent of uterine battles and pain. It is a jagged, unshaven landscape full of stretch marks and cowardly veins that collapsed under pregnancy weight. Mine is a body that managed a labor without contractions and the darkness of postpartum depression, as the light of my first child was brought into the world on a hot July day. I rocked this body around the bed, unable to loosen it free of panic, but kept it close to my child so that no matter what was breaking inside me, I'd keep him whole.

My body is a mother's body. It is not a dancer's body with perfect posture and well-shaped legs. Mine is a body that knows what an obsession dance can be but that movement no longer comes first. Though it responds to an inviting embrace of the Argentine tango, it does so with a reluctant and bothered ankle, broken weeks before the light of my second child was brought into the world on the day I, too, was born just twenty-five years prior. I crumbled under my own pressure, onto a mailbox at the corner of Kings Highway and West Eighth Street in Brooklyn. Cursing, I hopped home thinking that to labor with a broken limb is just what I needed.

My body is a mother's body. It is not my mother's body, with frail shoulders and cheeks full of Botox. Mine is a body of risks, piercings and tattoo ink. When the light is right and the mirror is bribed, I can see what my lover finds gorgeous. And though I claw at my body because it does not always make sense to me, I remember how bravely it got me through my only labor without pain meds, as the light of my third child was rushed into the world at the Brooklyn Birthing Center. He was the biggest baby ever born to those midwives, and he was magic.

My body is a mother's body. It was a "geriatric pregnancy" body when I carried my fourth child, a product of three queer people and a reciprocal in vitro fertilization procedure. It was a body healing from grief after my wife and I lost her pregnancy at twenty-four weeks, lucky to be in New York so that she could have a D&C procedure. It was a non-binary, agender body when I gave birth at home surrounded by people who knew without a doubt that my body was capable of more than I had ever thought possible. When I now feel my body, I know that my body is a mother's body and is well worth the worship.

There is nothing like a slurred "You're so sexy, baby" from some guy on the street to remind me that I am seen as a woman despite holding an agender identity. Even men who aren't strangers have said that I am "so obviously a woman" because I turn them on. Such experiences of sexism, laced with homophobia and racism when I am with my Black female partner, make it obvious that my struggle around gender takes a back seat to our collective struggle as people of marginalized gender and sexual identities, trying to navigate a world where white, cisgender, and heterosexual men hold a significant amount of power.

Shortly before my second was born, I began to struggle with the category of "woman" into which I was born and raised. Once I admitted to myself that I could not finish the sentence "I'm a woman because..." and explored identities beyond the gender binary, I was able to more fiercely carve out a safe space for my children. I must face how my own mother shaped my ideas of womanhood.

My mother's main lesson was that one's power as a woman comes from seducing men and appealing to the heterosexual male gaze, in addition to becoming a mother and a wife. Whether it was because our family is Russian Armenian or because the prevailing attitude across most cultures is one of patriarchy does not matter now. When I showed interest in taking charge of my pleasure or being with women, she took me to see a psychiatrist. When, at twelve, I came out as bisexual, the closest word I knew at the time to describe being attracted to more than just men, she cried. When I married at twenty, she was glad, hoping it had all been a phase.

Rather immediately, I became obsessed with getting pregnant, since that meant "having it all." Three years later, I was a mother of an eight-month-old child, banished from my house for leaving my husband. I was in love with another man, someone who was my equal. My new partner supported my being queer, the label I took up during college, and my exploration of gender. When we married, I was pregnant and determined to raise this child differently. As I became more involved in LGBTQ scholarship and activism, I struggled with my gender identity, and it took about three years to publicly come out as gender non-conforming, during a panel on transgender identities. It was a fleeting moment of being true to myself in a public setting, since without constant coming out, no one can "tell" I am not a woman.

I have to come out again and again because it never quite sinks in and some people simply forget that I am agender or that my pronouns are they/them. Generally, I never correct people if they use she/her, because I am glad to align myself with women and do, to a large extent, experience the world as women do. Though I would like to not be perceived as any gender, changing my physical appearance was never essential—I do not want to change my body, just the way others link it to womanhood. Not making a physical transition makes it difficult for people to see me as agender.

Even though mothering, to me, does not mean I'm a woman, it adds to my invisibility as an agender person because of the assumption that if one has been pregnant and birthed four children, they are even more of a woman. It is as if the assumed gender of my children helped solidify my womanhood, when to me, it undoes it.

Instead of being groomed to be "real men," my kids are raised free of gender norms, which allows them to develop their identities safely as they learn more and more about the world. And, prior to learning about gender, each of them gives me a gift. As an agender person, moments when I am not gendered are essential to my well-being and how I see myself, but they are rare. When my children are young, they are able to see me as Simone or Mommy without gendering me or seeing me as different from them. Even when they have noticed physical differences between their bodies and mine, I have explained everything from menstruation to genital shape without attaching biology to gender.

So when my kids look at me during those early years, their eyes are a place of freedom. In a way, motherhood has given me a way to find moments of validation for my agender identity, even if they are short-lived. I cannot say enough of these transformative experiences, because I know what it feels like when a person with no preconceived notions of gender is able to see the real me. I am an agender mother, and that is not a contradiction.

Conversation: Advice and Information

Solicited advice! Do you have any advice for trans, nonbinary, and gender-expansive people who are pregnant or want to become pregnant?

Aakash Kishore: This is such a big question. I would say you need people who really see you, who will honor and validate the path you are walking, who are committed to walking alongside you, who can be a soft place to land. In my experience, the pregnancy world in the US is very cis, white woman–focused, and even the way those women are cared for in health care and in society needs so much improvement. But there's also a degree of visibility and acknowledgment for the seasons of pregnancy and motherhood that doesn't broadly exist for TNBGE gestational parents. Instead, we face a season of invisibility and erasure while simultaneously working to grow life (and sometimes while also coping with unspeakable loss). When one of my neighbors started showing in her second trimester, other neighbors took immediate interest, asked after her, monitoring her needs, and bringing over food and gifts for her and the baby. The first acknowledgment for my family came well after bringing home my living child, and all queries were directed toward my wife; in eighteen months I had been visibly pregnant twice, given birth twice, gone through two postpartum recoveries, named two children, and released the ashes of one, without a single neighbor knowing to ask after me. There's no built-in "You've got this, Mama!" equivalent for TNBGE gestational parents. So we have to build our own.

Accessing even basic care as a trans pregnant person can be exhausting and demeaning. Having someplace where you can not only exhale but feel supported and empowered is so needed. Maybe this is with partner(s) or with chosen family or friends, perhaps it can be with a provider who is truly committed to TNBGE care, or it might be through online support groups. Wherever it is, you need and deserve connection, you need and deserve people, and you especially need folks who are committed to finding and sharing information, who can help support an empowered pregnancy and birth, no matter the outcome. What you are doing is too important to go at it alone.

Zillah Rose: Every now and then my kid will say they have a mom, and I will ask who that is and then tell them I'm not a mom. I then ask them if they know who I am, and of course they say my chosen parent word. Then I'll reinforce how all families are different. Some people have dad/s, some have mom/s, some have both, and some have neither, like us. We have no mom and no dad, and we are really an awesome, loving family. Even though I'm not married, and I don't have a partner or co-parent, we are complete.

My kid is recognizing that we are not like most of their peers.

Lots of observation is happening and that's okay!

Kids want reassurance. They need to feel secure in where they're coming from.

I take this time to change the mental-emotional patterns that I was taught as a child and took years to unpack as an adult. For example, one of my parents had a lot of self-image body shaming and low self-esteem for many years, and it really bothered me as a kiddo and then I adopted those insecurities. So now with my child, when they see my moles, rolls, chin hairs, and warts—the majority came with and got amplified with pregnancy and postpartum—I tell them, "All bodies are cool bodies."

"All families are cool families."

"Our family is a cool family."

I'm an older parent so not only am I mistaken as a mom, but I'm also often called grandma. (I'd much rather be called a dad or grandad!) I want my child to see and observe me being strong in knowing who I am and saying, "No thank you, this is my parent name and what my child calls me." I let my child know they're allowed to correct an adult or another child and be the teacher. Empowering our kids to be secure in our language of acceptance will roll over into other areas of life as they grow.

When I learned of my successful parenthood to be, I leaned into that I am going to be raising another human in a predominantly cis-heteronormative community as a solo genderqueer parent, and I was not going to go lie to myself, as for the rest of my life I'll need to deal with my gender dysphoria going up another level. How very true that was and is.

So my advice is thinking about how you would handle being called the wrong parent pronoun (by doctors, teachers, other parents, advertisements, store clerks, other children, the list goes on), if that applies. How will you empower yourself to become strong and set an example for your child? What if your child calls you the wrong syllable sound while they're learning how to talk, and if it lasts for months, what is your self-care plan? How will you reinforce that your family is beautiful as your family is and trust the process?

I found joining support groups on social media to be a safe space to ask questions or to release hardship. If able, in my opinion, joining an (online) parenting group or attending a Friday Zoom movie night with friends (who have/had kids) will really help the isolation one can feel through the last few months of pregnancy and first year of being a parent. I mention Zoom and online over going in person because of my own personal accessibility, but of course, attend in person if called to.

Having a place to be a person too is so important. For example, I used talk therapy every other week. For me, at times, this is where I get to be myself and not just a parent, housekeeper, yard keeper, homework helper, other job doer—hi, I'm a person under all those roles. I found having an established therapist during pregnancy was a good way for me to find the right match for when the baby came along, and adding anything new post-birth would have been too stressful.

I cannot stress self-care enough.

Kara Johnson Martone: One of the things I would do differently, as I look back on my choices and process, would be to do some real research about queer conception and pregnancy options. I didn't even realize there were other options, and we were pointed pretty quickly by my ob-gyn down the fertility clinic route. It wasn't until I got connected with our doula (at about six months of pregnancy) that there were resources and options for approaching family planning with a nontraditional lease. Even if we had ended up making the same decision about how to get pregnant, I wish that decision could have been made from an empowered and informed place instead of a place of desperation and confusion.

So I guess my advice would be to connect with some of the queer educators, doulas, and midwives in the community. Utilize Instagram and social media, literature, and anything you can get your hands on to find the queer folks making family planning accessible, inclusive, and empowering. Make family planning your own queer journey!

Tom: Last night, I had a dream about being late to a meetup with my friend. The walk we had planned was for 5:30 a.m. In the dream, my alarm didn't go off, the sleep was restful and deep. When I woke to the sun shining, I had an awful feeling of dread. In the dream I began picking up things in the room randomly and in a tantrum throwing things in the room—the lamp shattered, artwork smashed, and chairs flung aside that left holes in the walls. I was enraged about being late, about not being perfect, about missing this meeting that I had "planned for weeks."

When I woke, with my alarm as planned and the pitter-patter of Seattle rain outside my window and the smell of damp leaves, I listened for any resemblance of my dream, darkness still fallen, streetlights my only guide. That morning, I didn't miss my friend's visit, but my friend in fact forgot about our meetup, later explained through text. I found myself calm and generally content with the whole matter. I used the morning instead to write this response. Perfection and timeliness came up a lot throughout my pregnancy and birth, but I think that was because I forgot to dream. Dream about what it could mean and what was possible outside of what I continued to see around me.

Take some time to listen to your intuition, dreams, and visions about pregnancy and birth. Those visions have been lost to the systems of oppression (capitalism, racism, the gender binary . . .). Take pause and find pleasure in your dreaming—you are worth it.

Simon Knaphus: Right now I'm working on being sweet and kind to myself, on giving myself the love and support and affirmation that I hope I also give to the other people I am close to. I'm trying to be a good friend to myself! This doesn't mean dodging accountability or not taking an honest look at areas where I want to improve or am having a negative impact. It does mean giving my inner critic less attention than my inner friend and noticing when the unkind voice in my head is just parroting messages from systems of oppression. I would love to encourage others to be kind and sweet and gentle with themselves. I think that this is especially important when we are trans, nonbinary, or gender-expansive, and especially important when we are pregnant or trying to be, and especially important when we are parents.

I agree so much with what others have said. One thing that I keep coming back to when thinking about this is the importance of community. The friends and family members who were there for support, celebration, and just to be with on life's journey have shaped my experiences with pregnancy and helped them to be profoundly positive even when devastating. My amazing midwife really saw me and wanted to understand me and help me understand my unique pregnancies. My advice there is just to look for and nurture relationships with wonderful people, including care providers. Don't settle for people who treat you badly or make you doubt your worth. And when you're going through hard times, talk to the people who care about you—they want to be there for you.

Amber Hickey: Of my group of close friends who have given birth, I am the only person who did not have a traumatic experience. The birth of my first kiddo was not "perfect" or as I envisioned it, but I was very intentional about building a support network that ended up being crucial to preventing trauma/harm during the process. I wrote a bit more about this in my contribution to the book, but what I will say here is that I would recommend prioritizing building community around your birth (other pregnant people, a rad doula, skilled and sensitive providers, etc.). Also, be open to possibilities that are not aligned with your vision of the "perfect" birth. Try to listen to your body, as well as your little one and what is right for them.

My first baby was breech. I had been training (really, training!) for a "natural" birth since the start of my pregnancy. My partner and I had put hours into hippie breathing exercises. Giving birth is badass and I wanted to have what I thought was the full experience. I met with an OB to discuss ECV, a procedure in which a breech baby is turned manually to a head-down position. When the OB touched my stomach (in a way that felt uncomfortably firm), I had the immediate sense that ECV was not the right decision for us. I also had the sense that my baby would not respond well to it. I spoke with our doula, who provided additional guidance and information about how to have a C-section birth that felt as right as possible. We scheduled a C-section and are so glad we did. It turns out that our baby's umbilical cord was quite short. ECV might have disturbed the umbilical cord in such a way that would have required an emergency C-section, which would have felt a lot different than the calm, planned C-section that we had. Now I know that C-sections are just as badass (and just as natural)!

Edit after second birth: I did have a pretty traumatic experience this time, unfortunately. Rereading my entry above, I am worried that it sounds like I think my first experience of giving birth was not traumatic because of the community I had built around the birth. I definitely don't think that trauma can always be avoided, especially given the varied conditions we are all living in. But I am very thankful, yet again, for radical birth workers and the networks they build around them. They have been integral to the process of healing from the harm I experienced in January.

Kathy Slaughter: It's very lovely to read the previous contributions. Enthusiastically second the very essential need to connect with others and build support around you. Pregnancy is intense and magical, even when it's "easy" like mine. Never settle for people who treat you poorly, even and especially among your medical providers. There are true allies out there, or at least people eager to learn how to support you.

It is important to speak up about your needs and who you are. Many folks get lost in the emerging identity of "parent" and the all-encompassing experience of pregnancy. For me, it was even easier to lose touch with myself, lose myself, as a non-binary person. Even with loads of support!

TL;DR: Surround yourself with people who support you as an individual and your pregnancy.

g k somers: I also loved reading the above responses. For me, it comes down to listening to, learning, and knowing your body, mapping out the constellation of supports (community, family, etc.), and being ready to grieve. No matter how ready you are/think you are, there are likely aspects of your life that you will grieve.

As a non-binary trans person, I got to a place in my medical transition that really allowed me to feel ready to step into pregnancy. What I mean by this is that no matter how the world perceived me, what they called me, how they treated me, I was comfortable with myself. And I also knew that being pregnant would not make me a "woman" any more than being able to grow facial hair would make me a "man."

I spent years thinking about pregnancy, but that journey really only began once I started to take steps to live in my body comfortably (HRT, top surgery). Once I decided to actually try getting pregnant, everything happened really quickly. I did an at-home DIY self-insemination with help from a friend. We had discussed the possibility over the years and went through a questionnaire to make sure we were on the same page. (I didn't want a co-parent; he didn't want to be a father. I wanted to know that my kid could grow up knowing and connect with their genetic other half; he was open to getting to know my kid as my kid grew.) I got pregnant on the first try, and then it was all of a sudden like, okay, go time.

I worked to align everything in my life with the timeline of bringing this kiddo into the world—housing, school, work, finances—all while knowing that there would never be a perfect time, just the right time for me/us. I mapped out a constellation of all the kinds of supports I would need both during pregnancy and during the first year or so of kiddo's life (logistical, practical, emotional, etc.) and then made a long list of all the people in my life who I imagined might contribute in some way. Then, in the spirit of consent, I started reaching out to the people on that list and asking how they might like to be involved (e.g., bringing me meals when I was pregnant, or in aftercare, different types of emotional support, helping pick up baby supplies, childcare so that I could shower and take time to myself . . . this list goes on). It was really wonderful to see and acknowledge that while I didn't have a partner going into this process and wasn't going to be relying on the cis/het/monogamous/nuclear family structure that our dominant society upholds, I was able to create something that felt so much more robust and connected to my values.

Let's talk fashion! What did you wear?

Simon: My absolute favorite later-in-pregnancy clothes were oversized black overalls. I wore them most every day, even to work as a lawyer. I still wear them—I actually finally had to get a replacement pair when my youngest was about ten. I wore them with big T-shirts. As time went on, I switched to a couple of plain black T-shirts I got in the pregnant section at a big-box store, and sweaters on colder days. I also had two pairs of pants from the pregnant section—one that was gray with pinstripes and a wide elastic under-the-belly waistband, which I could wear with a sweater for a passably professional look when I needed that drag. The other pair were brown corduroy. They had the kind of adjustable elastic-and-buttons setup that pants for little kids have. They were really comfy.

Both times I stopped binding in the second trimester because it got to where it was more physically uncomfortable to bind than it was emotionally uncomfortable not to. I got a couple of what I called "sports tops." Those also got me through mammal-feeding—I would wear one under an A-shirt with a button-down on top. I could button down my outer layer and lift up my two under layers to feed my babies in a way that didn't show much of my chest, and I didn't feel the need to cover up with a blanket or anything. I felt awesome about feeding my babies wherever we happened to be, and with the clothing setup I felt like I was being myself.

One thing I didn't expect to need was pregnancy shoes! With my second, my feet got *so* swollen toward the end! I could barely squeeze into my flip-flops. If I could go back in time, I would convince myself to at least get some big slides or something else I could wear with socks so that my feet wouldn't freeze when I went outside.

Aakash: I totally agree about the slides. I got some in my second pregnancy and was so glad I did, but forgot to bring them to the hospital in the flurry of my water breaking six weeks early. Definitely wish I had them in those early postpartum days while my baby was in the NICU, because my feet swelled quite a bit more in those first seventy-two hours after giving birth.

In terms of other fashion, I wore joggers with the occasional sarong (at home). And I bought a couple T-shirts a size up, but wore my usual button-downs, flannels, and overshirts on top of those, just leaving them however open they needed to be to accommodate my belly.

Assuming nothing is TMI here, my bigger challenge was actually underwear/absorbency with the amount of discharge created by the nightly progesterone suppositories in my second pregnancy. It was both physically uncomfortable and emotionally triggering, and I was told by my provider to use panty liners, which felt particularly dysphoric at the time. I spent a *lot* of time online one week, first looking at menstrual underwear and then at incontinence underwear before deciding to just go with cotton Hanes boxer briefs because there's an extra layer of fabric that made them work better than my more environmentally friendly brand of underwear.

Amber: Pregnant or not, overalls are always the answer. Plus, a really nice robe, soft socks, and slippers for after you give birth.

g k: Absolutely overalls the entire first trimester and half of the second. Then I shifted into a Utilikilt and loose tank tops for the second half of my pregnancy, which spanned spring/summer months. I live near the beach, so summer mostly had me in swim trunks and shirtless, which definitely caused confusion with some of the locals, but hey. I rocked it.

Simon Knaphus

Placenta

The placenta is an organ, and when it's being cooked it really smells like one, like liver and blood. When my oldest was one month old, I cooked our placenta and the thick iron stench was so strong my dog went to the farthest corner of the apartment to get away from it. It was one of those days when you're like, "Fuck, how is it this cold?" We opened the windows to air out the apartment anyway. We turned on fans. I layered my baby in sweaters and a coat and blankets, then bundled myself up and went back to the stove. I added mushrooms, onions, garlic, and peppers, thinking I'd mask the taste. I didn't know how to cook meat and I didn't know how to cut it either. I've been vegan since I was a teenager. I didn't know what to do with the tough, stretchy membrane and cord on the one side and gnarl of blood vessels and flesh that was the rest of it, only partially thawed. With a dull knife and freezing fingers, I somehow divided it up into the pile of bite-size pieces that were later browning and sizzling, the wrongness of their scent screaming out that this was a very bad idea. My little one slept in a bouncy chair on the table while I heated up tortillas and brought the whole mess over. The other thing about placentas is that they are large. I sat with the local gay newspaper and my mountain of the worst food I've ever made and tried not to look at the bites, not to gag. I got full and fuller and uncomfortably stuffed, but I was determined, so I just kept eating. I didn't want to treat it like waste, this extraordinary organ, this connection between me and him. I wanted to turn it back into my body and offer it to him through my milk. I loved that placenta, and I had a plan for it.

Pregnant with my first, I worried about placenta previa—a rare condition in which the placenta covers the opening of the uterus and makes vaginal birth impossible. I didn't worry about the pain. (Thought I'd have an orgasmic birth—ha!) I didn't worry about me or my baby being healthy; I had faith everything would go just fine, except that placenta, taking root too low and expanding, inching its way across the exit. I did worry about one other thing. I worried I would be hit by a car and he would get hurt. I was so careful crossing streets. That was my first taste of the clenching fear that harm could come to my children.

Gender

Pregnancy is the most stereotypically masculine experience I've had. I was smelly and unapologetic and horny and strong and protective. I was impressively gassy. I dressed purely for comfort. I shed any remaining sexual currency I had retained as a not-really-passing FTM. I wore my body differently, performed gender differently, felt full of fatherhood. I was transitioning from a guy to a dad, which is part of fulfilling the normative male narrative. I was still flamboyantly queer, but there was a little bit of butch coming to roost. My gender identity stayed the same, but my experience of maleness broadened. I was shocked at how much I felt like Homer Simpson. I did not expect that from pregnancy.

I was afraid one of the people in my midwifery team would call me "her" while I was in labor, and my emotional reaction would interfere with my ability to give birth. I thought I would be going along naturally and "her" would trigger my cervix to snap shut like some angry sea creature and I would be forced to rush off to the hospital for a C-section.

My babies' genders: Of course, I wouldn't know anything about their genders until they told me, but there was a decision to be made about learning what their body parts were. I had a different partner for each baby. With my first, we decided to learn if he was an "innie" or an "outie" by ultrasound. We told everyone before he was born, thinking that when he was born the excitement of "He's here!" would be preferable to "Baby has a gender!" Before I was even pregnant, we had names picked out, and after we had the ultrasound, we announced his name and pronouns. That worked out just fine.

With my second, we waited to learn about his bits until he was born. We also waited until we met him to give him a name. We each came up with our own list of names and kept them secret from each other. I had a spreadsheet, because that's how I am. We loved the names each other had chosen for him, so he ended up with two first names, two middle names, and a hyphenated last name. That worked out just fine too.

T

Testosterone offered the promise of passing; it was a rite of passage and a means to craft the body and gender I was unraveling, or building, or discovering. I just needed to find some reassurance that T wouldn't cause problems for my future children. Because of my general preferences, the chances I would end up with a partner with a uterus who wanted to be pregnant were pretty slim, about as slim as the chances I would qualify to adopt. Plus, I wanted to carry, birth, and feed my babies. I yearned to take T, but I had to find out first if it would interfere with making babies.

I was fortunate to transition after the internet had started to really get going. I had the luxury of blog after blog, Friendster, the Binder Exchange. I learned testosterone would stop me from ovulating, so I wouldn't get pregnant on T, but that it's also not considered a reliable form of birth control. Nothing anywhere could tell me that if I took T and then later had babies, my babies wouldn't be impacted, so I didn't take T. I waited and watched for any study or breakthrough or story.

I moved to San Francisco, where I hoped to start T and have babies, the sooner the better for both! It was 2002 and then 2003 and I still couldn't find anything. None of my medical providers had ever heard of someone having a baby after being on T. My partner and I started trying for a baby. I sifted through the internet and found only one gem as I looked for anything about being trans and pregnant: someone suggested I email Matt Rice, who'd had a baby after being on T. I did, and he wrote a long, thoughtful response I am still grateful for. I can't get into my old email account, but I can feel myself reading it—encouraged that people like me can do this, my dream of being a parent starting to come true. I joined a listserv for trans parents and quickly learned that even in the trans community, in 2003, being FTM and wanting to be pregnant was not approved of. Oh well!

My partner was on T, and once, when I was sure I wasn't pregnant, I took a dose. I was antsy for our baby, but also for T. It was taking so long! I began to feel like it wasn't going to happen. Months later I was going to take another shot of T, but I figured I should take a pregnancy test first, even though I'd had several negative tests in the week before and was just about to start my period. It was positive! I called the midwife's office, and they congratulated me and signed me up for an orientation.

The Path

From an early age, I knew I wanted kids young. I wanted more of my life with them, more energy, and to be less old and out of it than my parents were. I figured out in my teens (it occurred to me when I was tripping on mushrooms) that my parents were actually very cool, and also that being a "with-it" parent didn't mean anything substantial to me. I grew up in Utah, where having babies young was what conservatives did. I grew up in a progressive household and was taught to follow my own path and to make my own reproductive choices. The assumption was that this meant having kids later in life, but I couldn't wait to meet them! When I was a kid and my family was setting off on a road trip, my dad would declare, "Let's get this show on the road!" That's how I felt about having kids.

When I was sixteen, I was in college and working as a nurse's assistant for a feminist gynecologist. I met and moved in with my fabulous boyfriend. We moved to Oregon and had a sweet queer domestic thing going. At nineteen I asked if we could start trying, but he wanted to wait until we were twenty-one. We broke up for other reasons (my fault), and I moved to San Francisco and got together with a trans guy who was great with kids and wanted to start a family too.

I was poor and young and trans and queer, and I never felt any of those things were reasons not to have children. It is never the logical time to have kids, at least where I find myself in history and culture. I don't have fields that need extra hands, and whether they take care of me when I'm old is entirely up to them. Having kids was a heart choice, completely. I was aware of the web of systems of oppression that would make things harder than they have to be, and I wasn't going to let those systems get in the way of what I knew was right for me. I was a queer punk and I was fine being an outsider; I had years of experience saying fuck you to oppressive norms and being creative about my self-expression. As a white person, this was less risky for me than for people of the global majority.

I read everything I could find: books and websites about getting pregnant, fetal development, radical parenting, queer families, healthy pregnancy, parenting babies, parenting toddlers. I lifted "mother" and "woman" from the page an inch or two, where the words hovered so there was space to add "father" and "man" and "parent" and "person." I understood why the books were written for women, and I didn't feel like I would fit most of my resources' target audience even if I were a woman, because I was a weirdo in many other ways.

By choosing to reproduce in the way I saw fit, I was bucking the prescribed narrative rather than complying with it. Most people are "supposed to" have kids, but I was the kind of person who is expected not to want to. I didn't expect to connect with parenting books, or with other parents, really. This wasn't something that bothered me. Rather than failing at a normal life, I was building a life that was right for me: robust, vibrant, ethical, challenging, and beautiful—at least most of the time. I found a midwifery practice where I could have an out-of-hospital birth covered by state insurance. I wore out the spine on *The Sears Baby Book*. We found and then changed donors.

Caregivers

The first time I gave birth was at a birth center that was not attached to a hospital. It was a home birth, but not at home. My insurance wouldn't cover home birth, and there was no way I could afford to pay for it myself. I was about six weeks pregnant when I went to the birth center for an orientation. I expected to meet a midwife with long, wavy, graying hair in flowy clothing who spoke with the slow warmth of a hippie grandma. Instead, I met Judi, a middle-aged woman who had short bleached and permed hair and who buzzed around and spoke with curt but caring authority. She wore a bright-blue swimsuit with pants and a fanny pack with a flip phone clipped to the strap, positioned across the top of her belly. Her eyeshadow matched her swimsuit perfectly. She had a few tics that would flitter through her fingers and lips while she spoke, which added more buzz to her energetic presence. She was more like a drag queen than an earth mama. I immediately adored her, trusted her as an expert on birth, and was a little concerned I wouldn't be able to relax into the process when it was time. When I was in labor and my baby's heart rate started to plummet, she grabbed my face in two hands, looked right in my eyes, and told me, "You need to give birth to this baby right now." This was exactly what I needed in order to do what felt impossible.

Her daughter Melissa was also a midwife at the birth center. I met Melissa at our intake appointment. She was wearing pajama pants and a Depeche Mode T-shirt. We ended up going way over our time because we instantly got along like old friends. She was excited to work with a pregnant trans person, not as a science project but because it was about damn time. She said she would do everything she could to educate herself and the rest of the birth center and encouraged me to let her know if there was ever anything I wanted done or said differently. She was the first person to hold both my babies on the outside. All told, it's been nineteen years and she's my person. We are going to go through each other's stuff after we die to get rid of anything we wouldn't want other people to see. Well, one of us is going to.

I was lucky to have another incredible support person, my doula and heart-friend Adriel. We met working at a health food store, and she still lives in that magical queer place between friends and family. Adriel doulaed me through pregnancies, miscarriage, two births, and a breakup. We were roommates when my oldest was little, and she became his aunt. Adriel was in her twenties like me, but the radical, magical earth mama style of love was already shining in her.

These three badass women are a major part of why I felt supported as a pregnant person, and they gave me confidence that I was doing great and would keep doing great once my babies were born. They were proud of me and loved my family. I wish this kind of care for every pregnant person.

Nuts and Bolts

When I was twenty-two, we found a sperm donor and started trying. For a year and a half, we lived in two-week cycles: waiting for ovulation, inseminating, waiting for pregnancy tests, bleeding, ovulating, inseminating, waiting. I cultivated a practice of not being pissed off that some people get pregnant by accident.

My first son, and a later pregnancy I lost to miscarriage, were made possible by a beloved friend who shared his sperm. I drew up a contract based on one I saw in a book for lesbians trying to get pregnant. It wasn't anything fancy, but I'm sure it would have held up if we needed it to. I tracked my ovulation by taking my temperature and sometimes using ovulation tests, but those were expensive! Especially on top of all the pregnancy tests I was buying. We used a cup and an oral medicine syringe (no needle). Sometimes we made a special occasion of it, and sometimes it was just routine. Eventually, twice, it worked. Like magic.

After the relationship with my first co-parent ended, I fell in love and became family with a cis man. Getting pregnant didn't take nearly as long!

Musings

People around me seemed more surprised that I chose to get pregnant than that I chose to transition. The underlying question was "Why would you take on that oppression?" For me, not having kids would have been bowing to oppression. Was it a political act? To use the body I was born with to pursue my gender, my sexuality, my family? Parts of life that are usually considered mundane, even compulsory. Was it political to have the audacity not to deny myself the full human experience? To live my own best life? I don't know if it had to be, but I think it was. I hope it was revolutionary.

I hadn't been near the process of pregnancy and babies. I think people in my community who had been closer to people with babies may have seen and accepted as inevitable the intense normalization process that new parents are sucked into like a whirlpool, both as a risk they were personally avoiding and as something I had inexplicably set myself up for. I have sometimes been exhausted by resisting assimilation: the forces of assimilation in pregnancy, the assumption that reproduction is assimilationist, the threat of my children being punished for my refusal to assimilate, the ways assimilation can creep in unconsciously, or is ceded to, under the many pressures it exerts. Also, I didn't go through all the work of being trans just to fit into another box, and what I've lost by resisting assimilation is tiny compared to the freedom I've kept. To be honest, I have assimilated in some ways. I don't swear nearly as much as I used to, my clothing is more normal (partly because I don't want people targeted by white supremacists to mistake my combat boots and cutoff camo pants as the opposite of what it means to me and to feel yet another threatening presence), and I'm more subtle about my sex life. I have middle-aged white dude drag for when we go camping in rural areas and for when I'm representing clients. Maybe this is aging, maybe it's thinking of others, maybe it's survival or cowardice—and probably some of it is assimilation.

Pregnancy and its institutions (midwifery, prenatal yoga, online spaces, birth classes) are places where women's knowledge and power have more room to breathe inside patriarchy, thanks to decades of feminist activist work. What did it mean for me to show up as a man expecting to have space in the room, a male voice of authority about my own body and family? Was I present as the oppressed (trans) or the oppressor (male)? Was I like the white person insisting on going to the BIPOC-only group? I knew that as a guest I needed to be aware of my impact and my manners. In addition to Adriel and Melissa, I found an online community of radical moms (shout-out to the Hip Mama blog folks!) who were just what I needed. We had those conversations, and we also talked about relationships and roller derby and tattoos and food stamps and toy weapons and music and everything else.

Feeling Pregnant

Before I was pregnant, I was excited about cuddling my baby for months inside my body, but after the reality set in, I wondered if I would feel as if an alien were invading my body, if I would be claustrophobic and want time to myself. Feeling my first baby start to flutter like a butterfly at about fifteen weeks, I forgot it had ever occurred to me. With both of my babies, imagining their little limbs learning what it is to be a body as they grew and got ready for personhood, I was so much more madly in love. I delighted in feeling our bodies sync together—times of rest and movement, how a walk or a ride would lull them to sleep, how they would get hiccups and then I would feel like I had hiccups because of their movements, how a smoothie would really get them going. (With my second, we sang Kimya Dawson's song "Smoothie" all the time, with slightly altered lyrics.) I was in law school when I was pregnant with my first, and I remember how he would get all fired up when I was debating with my classmates. I was representing clients when I was pregnant with my second, and his body raged with mine at the injustices they faced. Cravings were strong: My first wanted blueberry cornbread, and my second wanted chow mein and root beer.

Loss

When my oldest was about a year old, my partner and I started trying to conceive again. We were delighted when I became pregnant again after less time than the first had taken. I went to the midwife, and we heard the soft little heartbeat. We gave her a name. I held my hands over my belly and sent love to the little one beginning to form. I joined prenatal yoga. After twelve weeks we began to share our good news more widely, and then just two weeks later I started to bleed. At the hospital they did an ultrasound. I was having a miscarriage. I remember lying on the stretcher holding my belly so tight, as if I could hold her in. I howled, "My baby! My baby!"

We went home and I bled huge globs of congealed blood, I bled tissue, I bled through pads that looked like they were made for giants, blood leaked onto the carpet and the sheets. It ran down the shower drain like in a horror movie. My uterus clenched and squeezed and worked as uteruses do, and it felt like contractions, like birth way too soon. My toddler watched more movies during that time than any other in his life, because I just couldn't take care of him. It was probably only a week, but I remember it as the season I lost my baby. I still think of her sometimes; she would be about sixteen now. I used to mark her due date, but that place on the calendar has blessedly passed from my memory as the years have gone by.

Birth

My first was due January 11, but I wanted him to come a couple weeks early during winter break, because it seemed like the most reasonable use of time. Oh, the hubris! I took herbs to encourage labor, ate pineapple pizza from a place rumored to make people go into labor, spent hours on the swings at the park, pinched my nipples until they were sore, walked as much as I could, visualized going into labor—none of it worked. My partner wrote an eviction notice on my belly, and we baked two birthday cakes to convince the baby it was his birthday. It was probably because of these efforts that he was born only two days after his due date, on Friday the thirteenth, a dark and stormy night, the full moon. Actually, the perfect day.

Before going into labor, I thought I wanted to give birth in a giant tub and listen to *The Dark Side of the Moon*, because it felt mellow and like comfort food. During labor I got into the tub and couldn't really brace against anything. I felt like the bar of soap that can't be grabbed. Someone put on Pink Floyd, and labor stalled completely—it wasn't the right vibe. While they hauled me out of the tub, someone pretended the computer with the music was having problems, and we were suddenly singing along to "When I'm Sixty-Four" and labor was back on. He ended up being born to Beck's "Beautiful Way," which had come with my computer, because it was after the Beatles alphabetically. I didn't really know the song before, but I love it now.

My second was born to "Three Little Birds" two weeks after his due date. I agreed to Pitocin once it became clear the placenta was beginning to calcify. We planned to have a home birth at Melissa's house, because the birth center had closed and I didn't want to feel like I was hosting. We ended up being in a huge corner birth suite on the fifteenth floor of a hospital, perched high on a hill with views overlooking the Golden Gate *and* Bay Bridges! The sun set and rose and set again, glorious, but an unexpected reminder that time was passing differently outside our room.

The second time you give birth, it's supposed to be easier, but for me it was a lot harder. I was strong, and I sometimes found a peaceful oasis breathing and being fully present during contractions, but when I was thirty hours into labor and the Pitocin pains kept coming like a goddamn freight train and the epidural had me all distant from my body and I had even had the bliss of my first and only fentanyl high, I channeled my partner's strength, I imagined having his strength, and I pushed our giant, round-headed baby out of my body, and it was both impossible and the most natural thing in the world. He was my partner and my talisman, my anchor, the one who stayed awake when the drug gave me space to sleep. And when I woke, he was strong enough for the three of us, which was the most strength I had ever needed. The brilliant youngster grew in my body, but it was we who gave birth to him: my primal ancestral knowledge, our loving support people, and my partner's essential strength. Strength and love, vulnerability, and collective effort have been central to my experience. I have been a solo parent for thirteen years, but I have never been alone.

When I first saw my babies, it was like meeting a stranger who was part of myself. Their bodies were made of mine, but I didn't know their features, or what they thought. They're teenagers now, and I still look at them with awe. They somehow came from me, through magic and the most basic biology. I'm honored to have carried and birthed these two wonderful people.

Kathy Slaughter

My unexpected pregnancy came on the heels of my coming-out process. It wasn't the first time I'd ever talked about it, but it was definitely the most I'd ever honed in on my gender identity in my life.

You see, I have long questioned my gender identity to some degree—pretty much since I learned that was an option, in a very soft yet persistent kind of way.

It began in 2004 and 2005 in grad school, where my Intro to Women's Studies graduate class taught what would come to be called "queer theory" in the not-too-distant future. And I loved the idea of destroying categories. It made the most sense to me: that there was so much harm being done in our world because of the "normal" categories Western colonialism had created and enforced.

To me, the idea of just blowing these categories up was seductive, because I knew they created the ability for certain people to wield power over other people. And surely these categories caused so much pain and didn't really need to exist in the first place. Because everyone is such a unique individual. You drill down into the specifics and you'll find no two experiences are exactly alike, even with someone who's very similar to us, even when we resonate. Queerness was about defying categories, especially when it came to sexuality.

I hope my story resonates with other more quietly queer, genderqueer, non-binary people, people like me. But I am speaking my own truth about my own experiences and thoughts on gender. It is not meant in any way to dismiss or disrespect what gender means to someone else.

However, my view on categories has a pragmatic side. As I said, no two people are exactly alike in any way, shape, or form. Yet we are all also so incredibly similar, more alike than we are different. It is this knowledge of the distinctly individual differences and also broad similarities that, for me, creates this tension around useful categories versus unique individuals.

So the gender categories I most closely align with are non-binary and bigender. It's taken me a long time to find that language to understand myself more, for a few reasons. First, I am an elder millennial, and I grew up in a conservative family in a conservative state, in the middle of the United States. This was not a place where people were open about their sexuality in the '90s. This was not a place where gay was visible. Gay certainly existed here, and my community has always had a strong but hidden gay culture. It was hidden because it wasn't safe. And in these times in this state where I live, again, trans people especially are questioning safety.

It took me a long time to recognize that I felt more solidarity with trans experiences than I did with cis experiences. Part of why this was hard for me was because of how strongly the binary transgender people who I met throughout the aughts, in my twenties and early thirties, felt about their gender identity. Those binary trans people had a really strong conviction about who they were and what it meant to say that they were the opposite of the gender that was assigned to them at birth. And they had suffered so much because of this feeling that was so strong. Once they had words to articulate it, their experience was so clear and the categories obvious, whereas mine was more of a subtle "this doesn't quite fit" experience. But I have a lot of "doesn't quite fit" experiences in my life. So I didn't really notice this one per se. I focused more on other things, like practicing polyamory and being a social entrepreneur.

When I first learned about transgender, gender dysphoria was a clear requirement for being trans, a defining characteristic. Then partway through my adulthood, it was decided that was no longer true, that being trans was not defined by dysphoria. That was hard for me to really understand. I was so used to viewing dysphoria as The Thing that made one trans. Again, most of the samples I had seen of the trans experience were very strongly binary, while mine is a decidedly non-binary, genderqueer, woman experience, which has made it a bit more complex. And that meant it took longer to unfold. Once dysphoria was no longer a requirement, it gradually became easier to consider that maybe I was some kind of trans too.

So it hit me at the end of the pandemic shutdown. Like so many people, the time-out in the quiet of 2020 gave me space to ask some hard questions and to think things through. As that tragedy played out, I began to make some different choices about how I lived and how I expressed myself. I started asking people to use they/them pronouns with me. Then I went to my first festival in "guy mode," and I found it incredibly liberating to be seen through a more masculine lens. I felt more energy and comfort in my own skin.

About six weeks later, I found out I was pregnant, to my complete surprise.

So my pregnancy was defined by this experience of having my tender, more clearly defined gender identity almost immediately challenged by the woman-only, heavily femme experience of pregnancy. Part of me does truly feel grounded in the experience of womanhood. And that part of me felt thrilled to be enfolded into the lineage of mothers. Yet this masculinity that I had just begun to openly and fully express felt so threatened by it. I just didn't feel at ease.

Because of that intense discomfort, I am beginning to learn that while we must minimize our pain in order to keep going at times, it is incredibly important not to do it as a matter of habit. As useful as it can be to suppress how much of a struggle something is in order to get through it, it also means that you won't be very good at getting your needs met. The denial makes your needs harder to see.

Part of what made this so difficult for me is that I started the pregnancy experience without any fully established sense of what caused me pain or unease around gender stuff. I hadn't really interacted in spaces that weren't safe, that weren't supportive of the trans experience. And I was just completely unequipped to be abruptly dropped into this extremely singular gender universe that we call women's health care. Every book, every meditation, every support group, every class—with all too few exceptions, everything was about womanhood and motherhood and being connected to mothers of the past, present, and future. Mama this and The Mother that, and it didn't work for me. However, it also didn't hurt, because the most precise category I can currently give myself is bigender. I experience life with a foot in both camps of masculine and feminine. Like, this is stable, it's just me, and that's part of why my gender never felt that critical to me. I just relate to all of it. So it doesn't really hit that hard—like, yeah, it hurts, I don't love it because parts of me are being dissed, and it also doesn't slap how it does with my binary trans clients and friends. Part of me has been overlooked, and another part of me was like, yes, I feel validated, and I'm a part of this story. That cognitive dissonance is the internal problem, and it led to an intense struggle to belong. Belonging was influenced by me not being seen accurately as well.

Being seen accurately matters. That's why I use they/them pronouns: to ensure that the masculine side of me gets seen every once in a while. This isn't easy from a physical standpoint. I have a very curvy body, which means I have to work real hard to get at least as far as butch lesbian in appearance. And I'm still learning how to do that. At the time of my pregnancy, I had just decided that I was going to overhaul my entire wardrobe, as I hadn't really updated it since COVID and there was a gender shift to deal with.

Pregnancy immediately complicated how to deal with my appearance even more. Like, okay, I wasn't going to go buy a whole new wardrobe knowing my body was going to go through this morphing process for a year and who knows what kind of body I'd have on the other side. So I put off buying more clothes, because I had to. I did get some cute maternity clothes. But again, cute *maternity* clothes. Let's discuss trying to find cute, *masculine* maternity clothes. They don't really exist. Because my baby was due in the winter, I did find that buying extra-large men's flannel shirts was a fantastic solution in my third trimester and early maternity leave. Early parental leave. See, absolutely every word for everything related to birth and pregnancy has a feminine connotation built right into it. And I can handle some femininity. Lace and flowers are also things I adore. However, a constant onslaught of lace and flowers without some occasional, like, rough denim mixed in? Then I go a little crazy, because there's just a part of me that's like, *Hey, am I in the room here?*

It was also hard to really take care of that masculine side because I felt uncertain about moving closer to the seahorse dads, since I had this whole feminine streak going on. And I have a history of living through bi-erasure. To me, it seems like non-binary is kind of the gender identity equivalent to bisexual as a sexual orientation. It seems this way because I hear things like, "Oh, you don't really understand yet," or, "You haven't made your mind up. It's a matter of time. Clearly you're actually *this*." I've heard those same things as a non-binary person, just like I did as a bisexual person back in the day. So I was aware of the seahorse phenomenon. I knew there were trans men having amazing birth and pregnancy experiences. I wasn't sure if that was a community who would have welcomed me, either, because we do a lot of gatekeeping here in the LGBTQIA+ space. The alphabet mafia has a pecking order, and non-binary people are not that high up. So I appreciated the content. I got validation from seeing pregnant fathers on my TikTok feed, but I also didn't know if I could run over there and join.

Plus, as much as I was looking for community with other humans, I was also still questioning: Did I fit in this box? Remember, I don't like boxes; I don't want categories to limit the dynamic freedom of the individual. The label I would use exclusively if it was adequate still is *queer*. So I have this weird category/no category thing going on. And what it does is make it really hard for me to connect. I didn't know what the pain or discomfort was going to be like with each encounter, and so it just made me avoidant.

The avoidance impacted my attempts at education about pregnancy and labor. The mainstream resources recommended by my university hospital failed to be gender-neutral or gender-inclusive. I read what I could and enough to reduce my anxiety, and then I stopped looking. The friction was too much. Similarly, I never made it to the "trans and gestating" support group, even though the Zoom link was in my inbox every month. The mainstream resources that didn't even acknowledge gestating parents didn't work, and I wasn't sure what other spaces were welcoming for me. There were some inclusive offerings out in the world to learn about this whole pregnancy and labor process, but those were appallingly scarce. I found a few live classes, but none of them had things popping off during the window that I needed. Fortunately, I found one, exactly one, queer-focused, BIPOC-centered virtual course that I could watch anytime—Whole Body Pregnancy. This course was from a doula who was so wonderful with gender-inclusive language all the way through the program. Here I could engage, without needing to shield myself.

Finding these resources took me a while, because early in my pregnancy experience, like many newly gestating parents, I was just in my own world. I retreated a lot. It was me and the baby. I was starting to lean into that bond and my intuition, while also getting scared on the regular about miscarriage. I was slowly warming up to this whole idea, because this pregnancy was so unexpected. So I spent the first trimester just trying to adjust to everything. And then the second trimester I started taking in content, and it was just femme, feminine all the time, everywhere. It made me shut down. I was also minimizing my struggle rather than realizing I was struggling because the content was so woman-centric, triggering gender dysphoria. And since I couldn't admit to this struggle, it took longer for me to get my needs met. So I retreated. I got busy with work and with other things besides my pregnancy.

At the same time, I just enjoyed the physical sensations of it. I am definitely more connected to my body than I was before this experience—and I love that. It's such a beautiful thing, and it's a necessary consequence of pregnancy. I did not know exactly what my pelvic floor felt like before. Nine months of carrying a baby and having all seven layers cut through for a C-section I didn't want but ultimately needed forever altered my relationship with my own physical form for the better.

During my second trimester, I had no problems, as long as I just kept to myself. So I did. I was looking away from the difficulty that I was facing around gender, but my anxiety about getting some education and getting some support was growing. So that's when I finally broke down and told everyone on Facebook that I was pregnant and asked for help. I got connected to some Facebook groups that you can't search for because our safety is under threat. And I found a really queer-affirming, gentle, kind, supportive doula, who had some great resources from her training. I was her first genderqueer, non-binary client, so I knew that it was going to still be me finding the resources. But she also brought resources to me, and I was someone who was motivated to actually read them and listen to them.

My doula had created this cool labor meditation for pregnant women. And it was for women; it did not use gender-inclusive language. I listened to her original version, and I was like, *Oh yeah, this is fine. It's mostly first-person language that she uses, and the "mamas" aren't coming up too much. This isn't a big deal.* So I declined her offer to record it again, for me, using gender-inclusive language. I'm so grateful she didn't listen to me and instead said, "You know, I'm going to do it anyway, I think it's the right thing to do." So she recorded a gender-neutral version for me. I listened to it, and it was a night-and-day different experience than the first one, because I didn't have to filter or have my guard up against the references to womanhood. It was still essentially the same meditation, but simply shifting to gender-neutral language meant that I was not shielding myself from possible discomfort in order to get the nourishment.

My doula ended up being a surprise support in that way. And once I learned from that experience, thanks to the support of my therapist, who pointed out what I was dealing with, I went on a quest for an awesome curriculum. And I found the Whole Body Pregnancy. It's directed by a Black lesbian doula focused on being inclusive of queer people and centered on the BIPOC experience, Black in particular. That content was amazing, because I could take in the information about just how big my cervix was going to open, and what the pain was going to feel like, without having to protect myself from the gender-based discomfort.

My doula also connected me with this awesome podcast called *Masculine Birth Ritual*, which was a gender-expansive collection of pregnancy stories like mine. And it was an experience of pure gender euphoria, like a breath of fresh air. I only took in a few episodes, because podcasts are not my favorite platform. And yet I finally knew that I was truly not alone. And I had options. I learned about possibility models. I learned about giving people the information by posting it on your hospital room door. There are a lot of ways that you can assert yourself. And you can only assert yourself once you know where your pain points are.

I didn't have these affirming experiences until I was able to speak up for my needs. Which brings us back to my pronouns: Asking for they/them pronouns is a basic and simple way that I at least get the ball rolling on speaking up for my needs now. And from there, it just depends on the person I'm interacting with as to how they receive it. Is it something they're familiar with as an ally, or is it their lived experience? How do they speak to it? How do they respond? I learned so much nuance about the levels of comprehension and the ability to offer real help to me through this experience.

I'm so grateful for my partners' support around this whole evolution of my understanding of me. Through all of that, I found different ways to express my feelings. My first practices at asserting myself were through those closest to me, by simply sharing my truth. All three of my partners responded in affirming ways as my gender evolved, doing their best to change my pronouns when I asked. Each of them, as well as many good friends, noticed places where my story showed some queerness, affirming my understanding of myself. It gave me the strength I needed to assert myself outwardly as well.

With my partners, I could acknowledge the struggle. I used the resources from my doula to feed my creativity and help recognize my needs. One of my earliest assertions was my desire to use they/them pronouns for my baby, even after they were born. It seemed like the most natural thing to do. There is simply no way to know the gender of a baby. I can know the biological sex at birth, but their gender will emerge as they grow. It's like the next evolution of the "gender-neutral" parenting in the '80s. I can give my child as much space as they need to discover who they are, while also giving them a foundation of values and diverse formative life experiences.

By asserting this point of view with my child, we gained incredible, proactive support from the nurses at our hospital. Our child's gender is legally "unspecified" on their birth certificate. This potential outcome never occurred to me. In my conservative state, it's an option. Every single state agency employee has accepted it. My child will have the chance to define themselves in every possible way.

I've successfully avoided placing my child in a category, until we know more about who they are. Coming out of avoidance and facing all this discomfort and discrimination, acknowledging the struggle, enabled me to imagine what could be better. With the support and advocacy of my partners and friends—my chosen family—my child's gender is TBD.

Jamie Cayley

The Terrible Beginnings of a Beautiful Dream

Long ago, from as early as I can remember, I was certain of and at peace with the fact that I never wanted to have a child. I have very few memories about my childhood and teen years, but the ones I have are mostly filled with trauma, financial struggles, and a world full of unkindness. The systemic issues I have faced as someone who is transgender, neurodiverse, a person of color, and an immigrant made the world feel even more unkind. I did not understand why anyone would want to bring children into this world. And if I were to decide to raise a child, I would most definitely never choose to birth one. Or so I thought.

Everything changed when, nearing the end of my teens, I became pregnant during a particularly challenging period of domestic violence. Back then, I was on testosterone and believed my partner to be infertile. I had no way of knowing how long I'd been pregnant by the time I found out, and I had no safe way to access prenatal care. I spent months agonizing over what to do, because I knew that environment was not safe for me, let alone a child. I also knew I couldn't support a child alone. I was living in England at the time, and because of their citizenship laws, if I left my partner and had the baby alone, my child would not be eligible for British citizenship and would face many barriers. I knew I was running out of time to make a decision; it would soon be sixteen weeks since I had found out about my pregnancy, making the gestational age twenty weeks at minimum. I had been looking at clinics, but I kept putting it off, because even though I knew abortion was the only realistic choice that didn't end in predictable tragedy, I felt a strong bond with the baby from early on, despite all the fear, despite them being growing proof of my body being violated, despite all the exhaustion and horrible sickness I felt. I spent hours lying down feeling little flutters in my stomach and watching a bump grow, feeling little kicks, having conversations with it about all the things I couldn't tell anyone else, singing to it, trying to comfort it the way I wish someone would comfort me. I gave it a name: Addy.

But like all decisions starting from the lead-up to conception, I did not actually get to have a choice. I didn't get the chance to say goodbye on my terms. I had a stillbirth. I didn't even know it was happening until it was too late. I never even got to hold my baby.

I rarely discuss this experience, because many trans people believe that testosterone and estrogen and testosterone blockers are appropriate methods of birth control, especially in the long term. When I have talked to people about my experience, some don't believe me, because I was on testosterone at the time. I hear a lot in the media about how trans youth can't consent to hormone treatment because they don't have the maturity to consent to sterility, and I think it's important for people to know that going on testosterone doesn't necessarily make you sterile, even while you're on it. Many people, including trans people and so-called experts, believe that if a transmasculine person decides to carry a child voluntarily, they are not transgender, or they do not have gender dysphoria, and I have been told multiple times that any gender-affirming treatment will be discontinued or denied if I do not get a hysterectomy ASAP. I have also been refused testosterone indefinitely in the wake of new anti-trans legislation in Missouri due to being off testosterone for a prolonged period of time while trying to conceive. Most spaces for pregnancy loss only serve cisgender women and assume anyone who doesn't look the part is there as a partner, not someone with lived experience. Cisgender people, transgender people, doctors, and mental health professionals have all told me that if I was going to have an abortion on my own, I should have just gotten it over with—it's the same outcome. But how can they not get it? If you're stripped of your autonomy at every juncture, it's painful to have that last choice taken away too, even if the outcomes are "the same" and there's no clear culprit or explanation. I hadn't fully made up my mind, and I wanted a chance to say goodbye, but I lost the chance to make peace with the outcome and to have closure. However, as I've already hinted at by bringing up the impact that recent legislation in Missouri has had on me, that was only the beginning.

Having top surgery was the first step required for the second chapter in this story to begin. My dysphoria has always been primarily centered around my chest, so after the events that led to my realization that I want to carry and give to birth my own child, I knew there was no way I'd go through that voluntarily without having top surgery first. After my recovery from top surgery, as well as extensive therapy regarding the relationship that led to my pregnancy and that loss, multiple medical appointments, and years of saving, I finally felt like I was at a point in my life where I was ready to start trying to conceive.

I first had to spend six months off testosterone and start taking prenatal vitamins, per the recommendation of my ob-gyn. There were a lot of logistics and practicalities to discuss and for me to think through, because I am both aromantic and asexual and want to be a single parent, and because I am unwilling to entertain the possibility of "natural" conception methods. I considered using a known donor, but none are available in my friend group. There are apps to find "known donors," but I'm afraid I could end up in a custody battle with the donor if they have a change of heart about how involved they want to be. Due to discrimination in the system, I could lose custody of my child because I am trans, Latine, and only allowed to be in the country temporarily. Anything that could lead to a preventable and foreseeable risk of losing my child is not something that's a safe option—or that my anxiety and I could live with. That left using a sperm bank as the only remaining option, and with *Roe v. Wade* being overturned in the midst of me starting treatment, sperm costs have skyrocketed.

During the time I've been trying to conceive, I've had three different insurance plans with various levels of fertility coverage. My first insurance plan had the most comprehensive fertility coverage, but it also had a requirement that prior to starting treatment I had to be seen by a psychiatrist who is familiar with treating patients who are trying to conceive. I looked for a psychiatrist for two years but wasn't able to find someone comfortable seeing a patient who is trans and trying to conceive. That meant that I was only able to do fertility testing and at-home insemination with medication to induce ovulation. The medication was necessary because apparently I experience anovulation.

Once I got off the waitlist at another fertility clinic, I was able to start medicated IUI cycles while on my student insurance, which has no fertility benefits. Despite the clinic being known for having abundant experience treating transgender patients, I still experienced some issues with staff who seemed to be uncomfortable around me, along with someone changing my profile from transmasculine to transfeminine and accidentally erasing all my data in the process. While I was at the clinic, I had four medicated cycles, one of which was also ultrasound monitored. In total, since I started trying to conceive again, I've had two chemical pregnancies (a term for pregnancies detected around two weeks after ovulation, usually followed by a negative blood test shortly afterward) and two miscarriages.

One of the times I had a chemical pregnancy, I was sent to the ER for a suspected ectopic pregnancy, and despite being there for a whole sixteen hours, I was refused treatment and had to go in for an ultrasound at the clinic the following day after another sixteen hours of sitting in the ER waiting room. I have been denied accommodations at my university for fertility treatment, scans, and suspected ectopic pregnancies, and I have failed a class due to being late or absent because of appointments for IUIs or to have scans to verify I didn't have ectopic pregnancies, which led to me losing my practicum and being set behind a year.

Despite most of my income going toward covering a second insurance plan because it is supposed to provide IVF coverage, I have been denied coverage under appeal. Not only do I meet the plan requirements, the wait period, and conditions that allow the wait period to be waived, but I also have extensive genetic testing and karyotype testing because of my history of pregnancy loss and stillbirth. This should all make me eligible for coverage. However, on appeal the insurance company told me that I had no infertility factors and that because I am transgender and have been on hormones, I am considered to have undergone self-sterilization and will never be eligible for coverage. My doctors have not helped me appeal this decision. I likely would be infertile regardless of whether or not I transitioned, as it runs in my family and some of my diagnoses predate my transition. And as far as alternative funding options go, the funding program with the clinic costs less per month than my insurance does, but I am not eligible for it because I am not a US citizen or green card holder. Similarly, grants that fund IVF tend to require people to be in a couple, single cis women, and/or US citizens or green card holders.

It feels like all the odds are stacked against me, and some people tell me that if I can't afford IVF out of pocket, I shouldn't even be considering having a child. But here is what they fail to take into account: that I've spent all of my lifetime savings (around ten thousand dollars) on treatment and failed attempts to conceive; that living without testosterone when you're trans and being caught in a limbo where you have neither the hormones that make you feel human nor any idea if you'll ever be able to have the thing that makes it feel all worth it, even if it's only ever been fleeting, is the worst kind of hell; that I'd give anything for another chance to try even if it breaks off yet another piece of my heart, like all the previous times I thought it had worked and had to say goodbye too soon; and that my ovarian reserve matches that of someone who is forty years old or older, even though the testing was done when I had just turned twenty-four, so it's not like I have as much time as my chronological age would suggest.

Letters to the editor when comments about "irreversible fertility choices" being made by transgender youth were brought up as a reason to ban gender-affirming care throughout the legislative session were not published, and I was not allowed to give any testimony regarding that particular issue. I know that I would not be alive without gender-affirming care, and that I would not have felt comfortable carrying a pregnancy without having gender-affirming care first. If insurance companies were to expand coverage for fertility preservation for transgender youth, and not ban transgender adults from accessing fertility treatment, it wouldn't be the issue people are making it out to be.

But the worst people are the people who think they get it or act like they are supportive, only to use my journey trying to conceive as a reason to justify why I am a bad influence and stupid. Because no one in my life gets how isolating it is to be trans and deal with fertility treatment and pregnancy losses. To be aromantic and have no one else who is truly invested in the outcome like you are—the ups and downs, the joy and the heartbreak, all the little beings you named who never even made it long enough to have a detectable heartbeat. And the one who did, but you still couldn't ever hold regardless.

There's nothing in this world I've wanted more than to be a parent and carry my own child, and I am still determined to make that happen. But in the meantime, I hope to be able to turn the seahorse tattoo in my soul into one on my skin, one more declaration to the world that it cannot erase people like me.

Conversation: Pregnancy Care

Did your care providers have trans-, nonbinary-, or gender-expansive-specific knowledge or experience? Were you able to find providers who embraced your gender? If so, how? What advice do you have for people when interacting with pregnancy care providers?

Tom: I wish my care provider had inquired with me, but they just went ahead and provided care assuming my gender. At the time, I was only given two binary options to fill out the medical forms. I know there is slow movement to change this, but it's very sad and very common. Going based on the forms that I completed, my provider gave me the care she thought I had wanted, but what I wish someone would have done is stopped and asked, "What services or care are we not giving?" and found options and resources for me. I wish someone had paused and given me some space to talk about what I was feeling and experiencing about the changes in my body, but that isn't the job of health care providers that I had (but I wanted it to be). That was nine years ago.

Today, my GP and I had a very in-depth conversation about my gender. She gave me additional information, resources, and even asked for a more supportive, longer consultation. She happens to be at the same hospital where I gave birth, which baffles me. How did I find the provider that I did? I had to do a lot of research and asking around. I also expected some disappointment with the GPs that I did meet with. But I kept hopeful that a provider would be good for me. Like our earlier conversation on community and support, I asked for lots of help.

Aakash Kishore: The midwife I worked with most closely in my two pregnancies did not have previous experience working with trans clients. We had very different lived experiences, so there were times when she struggled to see the significance of certain things I went through as a pregnant trans person of color, but she was earnest, caring, and open to feedback. I don't know if this will make sense to anyone else, but there's a difference between someone trying to act "normal" around a trans person versus actually acting "normal." Like, sometimes you can see the gears turning in a person's head as they try to remember the thing they once learned about how to interact with a trans person? I never felt that way with her. She listened genuinely, was willing to look into resources and make calls on my behalf, and when there weren't good resources to offer, she was able to provide so much support in the form of empathy, validation, and a listening ear. She also treated me with dignity and wasn't afraid to touch my body—always asking for consent and then moving with ease, clarity, and purpose, and, like Tom said, was ready to dedicate more time when necessary. She's the first provider to perform a painless Pap on me and the only one to ever perform a chest exam.

The perinatologist who comanaged my care in my second pregnancy did have experience working with trans folks in some capacity. This was really important to me, because I had so many unanswerable questions about the cause of my cervical insufficiency. She knew the research, understood the gaps, and was able to extrapolate from the literature to help ease my fears that I had done something to cause it (particularly, that being on T for over a decade had played a role; it didn't). She also specialized in caring for pregnancy after loss. There were still some things she didn't get, but overall it was helpful that I could speak openly in our appointments about the range of experiences that were shaping my pregnancy.

I also worked regularly with a pelvic floor physical therapist and an acupuncturist who were both cis women of color who had experience or specialized focus in working with trans folks. Their caring touch was so important to me after having the hands of so many unsafe white folks on and inside me.

In terms of selecting a provider, consider that at some point you are going to be fairly naked in their presence. There's a high chance you will pee and/or poop in front of them. So if it doesn't feel comfortable to sit in an office fully clothed and have a conversation, or if your body doesn't feel safe when they lay hands on you, it may be pretty difficult for your body to relax and open up in the ways it often needs to when it's time to give birth. If the provider can't accept when they don't know something or if they center themself rather than you when they make a mistake, those might be indications to find a different provider. Having other supports as a part of your birth team can make a big difference too, especially if there are circumstances that limit which providers you can see. Having a support person in your appointments whom you trust to advocate for you can be very helpful, and hiring a doula who has worked with TNBGE folks may help create more safety during labor. I would also definitely recommend looking into other forms of caring touch (e.g., massage, physical therapy, acupuncture, chiropractor) as a part of a pregnancy care plan if you can access them. If you have insurance, certainly see what services are covered and take advantage of as much as you can.

Amber Hickey: I have had amazing queer doulas during both of my pregnancies. Purely by chance, I also had a supportive OB during my first pregnancy. For my second pregnancy, we are in a different location, so I asked a midwife which OB was most supportive of queer pregnant people and she directed me to the right person. So overall, I have had good experiences with care providers thus far. I will say that I decided to opt for an elective C-section this time—even though Baby is now in position—because I want to limit my interactions with the generally very religious staff at the hospital where we will have baby number two. A C-section feels more predictable in this case, though I am mourning the possibility of going into labor and giving birth without surgery and the tough recovery that will entail. (And of course, recovery can be tough regardless of how one gives birth!)

I would recommend beginning to advocate for yourself when you first fill out the paperwork at your health care center. For instance, during both of my pregnancies there has been nowhere to write my pronouns on the paperwork, so I have added them in the notes section, along with my preference not to be called "Mama." What you put in those forms should go in your chart, so every nurse, etc., will have access to that information. I also recommend finding a queer doula who can help you find tools to self-advocate, as well as be there during the birth to create the safest possible conditions for you and your family.

Edit after my second baby was born: My OB during this pregnancy was probably the most supportive of queer folx at that hospital, but I ended up having a terrible experience with her overall. If I could do it over again, I would also prioritize finding an OB who is committed to a trauma-informed approach. (I assumed she would be, but I was wrong.)

Kara Johnson Martone: Yes and no. We were originally working with an ob-gyn who routed us toward fertility clinics. And in that arena we did not experience much understanding of trans or queer families at all. Once we became pregnant, we sought out doulas and childbirth courses that were specifically trained to work with queer and trans families. This helped tremendously in understanding our rights and how to navigate the systems in ways that felt good for us.

My suggestion is to always do research first. There are queer birth workers out there who have so much beautiful and profound knowledge. Take the time to sit with the different options out there, and know that your experience as a queer person may lead you to less traditional means of existing in the world. Your needs and desires around childbirth and parenthood are valid and important, so take your time to sit with all the options and figure out what feels most in alignment with you.

Simon Knaphus: I second what folks have said about doing research and trusting your (adorable pregnant) gut. Yes, you're going to be naked, probably pooping, in front of this person! I only had one option for out-of-hospital birth covered by Medicaid, and I'm *so* lucky that I found my midwives and their birth center. They didn't have any previous experience with trans people, but they were informed allies and just felt right from the get-go. My doula was one of my best friends.

There is one thing that went sideways when I was pregnant with my younger son. The birth center had closed, and I was trying to get an exception from the insurance company so I could have a covered out-of-hospital birth again. I went to the OB my insurance company had assigned me to for this referral, without learning anything about him. I basically just needed him to sign a paper. Before the exam room, I went into his office, and the vibe was off. The walls had wood paneling, and there were what appeared to be painted portraits of his fancy little dogs. I could see that being campy and amazing, but with him behind the desk it just added to the David Lynch feeling. I explained my situation, and he told me he would sign the papers but he needed to do an exam first. I thought he would just need to confirm that I was pregnant with a pee test and listen to my belly, but he started messing with my nipples and then told me he was going to do a Pap test. (He called it a

"Pappy." Gross!) I knew from the first time around that there was no need for a pants-off exam until the final weeks of pregnancy, so I told him no, that I had a recent Pap test and didn't want another one. He got kinda huffy and that was that. The paperwork never worked out. Yeah, trust your gut!

g k somers: I have the privilege of living in a city where I was able to specifically seek out trans-affirming care throughout my pregnancy. I worked with a midwife team where one of the midwives was a non-binary gestational parent, so I really felt affirmed in that part of the process. The downside being that not everyone on the team was as trans competent, and one person on the medical team actually gave me some potentially harmful information. I questioned the information and then sought out a second opinion before proceeding from the non-binary midwife, who validated my suspicions. I'm really glad that I trusted my gut and sought out a second opinion, but in the moment, I was hella angry that one of my care providers gave me information that could have potentially led to a miscarriage. The information was around trying to induce lactation, but the information was meant for nongestational parents (i.e., trans or cis women who were not carrying).

I also worked with a non-binary doula who was a good friend of mine, and my entire birthing squad was either trans or non-binary. I advocated for a home birth (wanting to avoid hospitals, misgendering, sterile environments, etc.) and trusting my body. While my birth didn't go exactly as planned (a quick labour meant having to ditch the birthing pool and just go with birthing on the floor!), I'll say it went exactly as it was meant to.

Sam Vanbelle: I was part of a study in a hospital in Gent with a big gender care unit and a fertility clinic. They searched for persons who got gender and fertility care there. They also interviewed nurses and doctors. I was always very nervous for doctors and midwife appointments. But what struck me in this study is that the caregivers are also very stressed for appointments with trans people. Stressed about saying or doing the wrong thing, stressed some of these patients get angry. The time they get to give this care is quite limited, so some things they have to do on automatic pilot. The time limit makes it more difficult to create the headspace to give the appropriate care. This knowledge helped me to be more patient with caregivers. To instruct them gently on words you prefer, on ways you like your care. This openness from my side opened it up more on the other side and made more space for good care. I could leave behind a lot of anger about weird treatment moments. And although it may sound nonconfrontational, it helped me to be confrontational in a way that suited me. And if caregivers just don't want to listen, or are ignorant, it's never a bad idea to leave them behind and search for a better one, in the knowledge I live in a place where it's quite okay to be queer or trans.

Amber Hickey

Support Amidst the Hot Mess

My first pregnancy started in late 2020, during the height of the pandemic. I felt sick all day during my first trimester, but I still wanted to move, so I registered for a virtual prenatal yoga class.

"Hi, mamas!" the instructor greeted us from her beachfront home yoga studio in central California. I had not prepared myself for this immediate assumption of gender identity, even though looking back I suppose I should have. My body really needed some recuperation, but I ended up leaving that class feeling even more nauseous. Afterward, I started researching queer prenatal yoga classes, queer pregnancy groups, queer doulas—any resources that might feel more supportive than what I had just experienced.

Before I was pregnant, assumptions about my gender identity did not hit as hard as they did during pregnancy. Those assumptions and my encounters with them increased exponentially while I was pregnant. Thankfully, I was able to quickly connect with a rad doula, a supportive queer pregnancy group made up of mostly non-binary and trans folx, and an affirming team of providers. Even though I lived in a smaller, largely straight and cis town in Maine, the mostly virtual community of queer and queer pregnant folx who I intentionally built community with at that time were crucial to my largely positive experience during my first pregnancy and the birth of my kiddo.

Serendipitously, I also lived next door to a queer abolitionist birth worker, whom I could seek advice from at any time. She was also genuinely interested in hearing about my experiences and what I was learning in the queer pregnancy group. Even though she was already a friend, it felt good to sense that my perspective as a non-binary pregnant person really mattered to a provider. I truly do not know how things would have turned out without all of those amazing people, and I am grateful for the labor that queer doulas and providers have devoted to creating safer, more affirming spaces for queer pregnant people.

Now, in summer 2023, I am pregnant again—but this time, I live in Tennessee. It's difficult to put into words how it feels to be queer and pregnant here. My doula in Maine had to travel around an hour to meet me at the regional hospital closest to my town, but the closest doula to not assume that all pregnant people are women—or at least the closest one to have more open language on their website—to where I now live in Tennessee is two hours away. I asked the midwife I have been seeing which OBs at the hospital are queer friendly, and her list was exactly one person long. Anti-trans laws and anti-queer sentiment are gaining momentum so quickly in this state that I am increasingly fearful of how the fact that I am non-binary will affect my care and the care of my future kiddo—whom I do not plan on gendering. Not to mention the exodus of providers from this region since the *Dobbs* decision. I want to build connections with other queer pregnant people in the South, but I don't know where to start. So many folx have already left the area or are understandably guarded about their identity for fear of animosity and violence. I was also diagnosed with multiple sclerosis in December 2022, so I am trying to find ways to navigate how to advocate for gender-affirming and disability-justice-informed health care.

Despite all of these challenges, I am hoping to be able to translate my positive previous experience to this one—which is fast approaching. I witnessed my doula advocating for me during my first pregnancy, so perhaps I can be a better advocate for myself this time. I learned tips and tricks from queer doulas and pregnant folx: writing pronouns on a sign outside of your hospital door or on the whiteboard inside your room, delegating tasks (asking the provider to pass on the message to everyone else in the room not to announce the baby's sex), and making sure that the head nurse knows that under no condition do I want to be called "Mama." Honestly, I don't know if anything could be more difficult than getting certain relatives to understand that one, much less put it into practice. Not surprisingly, my kid has never called me "Mama." One of the other people in the pregnancy group I participated in told us that they were going to let their kid choose a name. I loved that idea and let my kid choose my name too. It's a super cute name—they did a good job.

Within all of this, it gives me joy to know that although my kiddo might always live under challenging political conditions, I have no doubt that they will be one of the people creating the supportive community that so many of us need amidst the hot mess. Sometimes when I am exhausted and just need to lie on the couch, my kid instinctively understands and nonjudgmentally knows that the only thing that will help is a good cuddle.

Kara Johnson Martone

Belonging and Transformation

To be born queer in this society is to be born with a tension between self and belonging. Many of us are born into families with siblings and parents who don't share our identities. I was aware of my differences fairly early in my life. This awareness caused me to develop a hyper-vigilance and overanalysis of others' behavior and sent me on a path of self-exploration and understanding. This is a story about a part of that path, a moment in the journey of my life, and how the memories of pregnancy and childbirth transformed and shaped my identity. This is a story about evolution and connecting with self. This is a story of how struggle forces this growth, and a story of the transformation that blossoms after living through difficult experiences.

There are some important things to know about me as you read through this story. I am a neurodivergent, queer educator and therapist. I have been working in human services and queer advocacy for over a decade. I am stubborn and optimistic, especially when confronted with a challenge. A former collegiate athlete, I relied on my body's strength and the power of my mental fortitude to push me when I faced a challenge. I had always been able to push my body to perform, and I believed that I could push myself to do anything.

What I didn't know was when to stop pushing. I never learned to listen to the mechanism that told me, "Stop, this is too much." I believed I was invincible, and in control of my life. I was fairly certain that I would handle any physical difficulties with ease. I had no concept of the privilege I had experienced, and I believed my body would do as it always had: put up and shut up.

Beyond my physical body, I am friendly, open, and have a witty sense of humor that has carried me through difficult situations. My humor and openness were great assets growing up in Colorado Springs, a small conservative town where I had felt like an outsider for as long as I could remember. I spent my youth fantasizing about the sweet ease of belonging and worked diligently to feel like I was a part of something, at great expense to myself. I spent my twenties trying to find that belonging in every queer bar in Denver.

At thirty-one years old, with my face still buried in a pitcher of beer, my partner walked into my life. Suddenly I felt that belonging. It was a U-Haul romance, moving in together after just a few months. As we continued building our life together, my desire to have a child grew. It was a paradoxical desire, to reach the pinnacle of freedom and independence just to give it all up.

I always dreamed of becoming a parent and having a little family. I fantasized about all the wonderful and magical moments. I fantasized about the connection, growth, and love I might experience in those moments with my own family. I dreamed of having a community to belong to and building that community with the family I created.

I was the first queer person I knew to vocalize that I wanted a kid. Much of my queer community was focused on developing their own identities and accessing long-sought-after liberation. When I talked about wanting a child, I was met with blank stares and grimacing eyebrows. Words like "breeder" and "normie" were used to describe my desires. I started to feel a disconnect with my queer community. I felt misunderstood, scared, and alone. The weight of the disapproval sat in my chest and pressed on my diaphragm, and it felt all too familiar. Once again, I didn't belong. This feeling was a nudge from the universe, a challenge to sync my body and soul. This was a chance to transform into the person I was becoming, a person I had no model for. This was a nudge to move forward into the dark.

With no idea how queer folks acquire a child, my partner and I started down a path created by and for heterosexual folks struggling to have children. We found ourselves in a fertility clinic, wondering if we were in the right place. Right away I knew we didn't belong. The year and a half spent at the fertility clinic was filled with moments of panic, missteps, overstepping, microaggressions, isolation, confusion, and a global pandemic. In these clinics and medical offices, I felt stripped of my queerness and freedom. I felt uninformed, disenfranchised, and incredibly out of control. For about six months, I was forced to out myself and my partner at every meeting. No one was aware of queer families, queer identities, or the needs of queer folks. There was no use of inclusive language or space for difference. Then exhaustion took over. I was too tired to fight the battle, to be every employee's first lesson, so I let myself be misunderstood.

In all the ways I felt alienated, my partner did more so. Their presence at the fertility clinic was rarely mandatory, their genetics unnecessary. They were scientifically insignificant. I began to feel disconnected from the one place I belonged. This was particularly upsetting to my partner, and it pressed like a knife on their own desire to belong. The pressure of being misunderstood had clear impacts on our relationship. Because we were both confronted with unique struggles in the process, the experience drove a wedge between us.

When most people think of childbirth, they naturally think of the word *push*. But in my experience, pushing started long before childbirth and even pregnancy. I pushed and pushed through the difficulties presented at the fertility clinic. I pushed through my partner's resistance and worries. I pushed through the stress that synthetic hormones placed on my body and the stress that my partner's graduate school tenure placed on our relationship. I pushed through a global pandemic and the pressure of providing a single income for our family. I started to reorient myself as a person who was perpetually under pressure; slowing down to assess the damage of these stressors was out of the question.

It was during this time, before I was even pregnant, that I committed to the idea that I would give birth at a birthing center. I wanted to experience the physicality of birth without the medical intervention. I wanted to experience the process and feel the birth happen. I believed my body was up for it, because my body had always responded positively to my pushing. Why would this be any different?

In February 2021, the day arrived. I was pregnant. I became pregnant quickly. Meaning one day I was not pregnant and the next day I was four weeks pregnant. This is to say our embryo implanted and became a successful pregnancy. Along with a quick pregnancy came quick morning sickness. Seemingly overnight, I was drained to my core, and only then did I begin to realize how the previous year spent pushing through injections, a changed body, and extreme pressures had compounded.

I began neglecting laundry, dishes, and any connection with community and friends. My usual bubbly, social personality slid into a void of energy that made it difficult to engage in anything. The optimism I've always been known to have slowly dried up, dulling my sense of reality except to feel pain and exhaustion. I began questioning so many of the things I had clung to as truths about myself. I had always been a happy and social person more prone to anxiety than depression. I now found myself struggling with prenatal depression, losing track of myself and fading into darkness.

One of the first problems I encountered with my pregnant body was understanding my limits—an awareness I hadn't needed until the height of my pregnancy. I was working full-time to provide the sole income for our household, going to family therapy with my parents, and fielding microaggressions at nearly every turn. In addition to the upheaval in my personal life, the world had just started to grapple with COVID-19 and the panic and stress that the pandemic had induced. My world felt like it existed in an immense pressure cooker. I believed I had no choice but to put my head down and block out the world to survive. I was no longer concerned with cultivating joy and connection.

As a therapist, I have based my life and education around the connection between mind, body, and spirit. Aligning these elements allows for a greater ease of life and an ability to navigate difficult situations. Contextual factors like oppression and struggle due to marginalized identities play a huge part in one's ability to access this alignment. My ability to remain balanced and in alignment had been pushed too far. The pressures of existence had become too much. My ease in life had disappeared, and instead I was focused only on survival. Looking back now, I see the immense pressures I carried as my body was growing a baby. Many of my physical symptoms were manifestations of my mental and emotional stress. My prenatal depression was caused by the slog of sickness, isolation, and overwhelm. I suffered constant stomach upset, nausea, and reflux. I started getting migraines and found it difficult to get out of bed.

At around the nine-month mark of my pregnancy, my partner told me that they were concerned for me and the baby. They pleaded with me to leave work two weeks before my due date to give myself time to rest and relax. They asked that I discontinue family therapy and shift focus to myself and the baby. It was well past time to prioritize myself and my health. I couldn't see it at the time, but this was a pivotal moment in my understanding of self. I was confronted with the reality that I did have a limit and that pushing beyond that limit was not healthy, beneficial, or even possible. I felt heartbroken and defeated knowing that this pregnancy would never be what I had dreamed.

The weeks between leaving work and the birth were incredibly slow. The days of sickness, desperation, and waiting felt eerily never-ending, like we were living in a twilight zone between our past and our future. Those weeks were filled with our favorite shows, hitting up the local nail salon, and taking short but frequent walks. We did our best to fight the seemingly endless slog.

Four days after our due date, I began having contractions. At around 6 a.m., I started to feel the sharp pain in my lower abdomen. I remembered the lessons from my doula and birthing classes. I got out my timer and started tracking space between contractions. I tried to count the minutes, but the harder I focused the more confused I became. My contractions would come and go, build and stop. Many hours went by like this. The wait was endless and the confusion constant. After eight hours, we decided to call the doula. Our doula worked with me and my contractions, my dogs lying by my side. We decided to head to the birthing center after nearly twelve hours of contractions. We entered the birthing center eager, hopeful, and terrified.

After thirty minutes, the midwife came to the room and discussed my marked decrease in contractions and slow progress. The odd contraction pattern had continued, building over time but stalling out periodically. The midwife shared with me that I was not ready to have the baby and that because they were a low-intervention birthing center, my contractions were not strong nor consistent enough for them to treat me at that time. The midwife suggested we return home and wait for more progress.

I was devastated. I was exhausted. I was confused. This was not how I thought things would unfold. I felt the air drain from the room as I was confronted with the reality that I would not be giving birth anytime soon. I had so desperately wanted to make this room my home, to bring this baby into the world. I wanted to feel held and safe. I wanted relief from the pain I had been experiencing for months. I was heartbroken and afraid and felt completely lost. My partner packed up my belongings and got me back in a wheelchair, and we headed for the car. In that moment, I felt another turning point that propelled me to come back to myself, after months of detachment.

The next day, the doula returned to our home as contractions started again. Twenty-four hours into labor, a different perspective and reality started to take shape. I was beyond exhausted. At around 6 p.m., the contractions started to build, so we decided to pack our bags and make a second attempt at the birthing center. Before stepping outside, I stopped my partner and doula at the door. I looked at them and said, "I'm not coming back here without a baby. I can't come home from the birth center again." They looked at me, nodding together, and said, "Okay!" That simple declaration of what I needed brought my body and my soul back in sync. I was aware of my needs and my limits. For the first time, I could feel my body and soul begin to collaborate. It was a powerful moment that propelled me into a new way of being.

We returned to the birthing center and were told that I was still not far enough along. At three centimeters dilated, there was nothing they could do for me. My partner and I sat in our room at the birthing center and made the decision to move to the midwife center located in the hospital across the street. We loaded up, once again. Me in the wheelchair, my partner the pack mule.

Check-in at the hospital was swift. I was hooked up to a series of monitors making sure the baby was safe. As they monitored the baby's heartbeat, they noticed the baby was under a lot of stress. After talking with the midwives, we decided it would be best to give my body some relief, and I made the decision to get an epidural. After over thirty hours of labor, I was exhausted and dehydrated and needed help.

I fell asleep and woke up six hours later. I had dilated to nine centimeters. The midwife came in and told us the baby's stress was increasing with my contractions. There was a possibility the baby was stuck and unable to move down the birthing canal. As we discussed the possibilities for birth, she looked me straight in the eye and said, "If you decide to go for a vaginal birth, you will need to push from the depths of your soul." I didn't even know what that meant. How could I push when I had hardly slept over the past twenty-four hours? I hadn't eaten in days, and I couldn't feel my body. I took a moment to think and process with my partner and doula. I decided the best decision for me and the baby was to have a cesarean section.

This was not the birth I had imagined. For weeks, I witnessed people giving birth via videos and Instagram posts. I saw queer couples give birth in their homes. I saw the community around them share the burden of trauma and excitement. I expected myself to operate outside the system, because I found my belonging outside the system. Yet here I was, face-to-face with the reality of my bodily limitations. We needed the system. We needed the very thing that oppressed us. I wanted so badly for my queerness to be validated in my birthing story. I wanted to connect with myself on a deeper level. Instead, I found that pregnancy and birth moved me so far away from myself that I was lost.

The C-section was one of the most traumatic memories of my life. After many days without sleep, and little to no food, I clung to my partner's arm under bright white hospital lights. I was terrified and wondering what was happening to my body. I was sick from exhaustion and the medications, throwing up into a baggie held to the side of my face. My body began to convulse. I would learn later that this is a normal side effect of the medications, but in that moment, I was terrified. I felt as though I was in a space between life and death. Riding an electric fence straddling this world and the next. I looked into my partner's eyes, and I learned what it was to truly be loved. They were my only comfort in the complete chaos. My safe place, and my home. In those moments, I felt deeply and profoundly loved. I learned in an instant that I am of great importance and that I am worth more than what I can push myself to do. I am so grateful for that knowledge and the feeling of love and connection while I simultaneously grieve at the lengths I had to go to in order to feel it.

After forty-eight hours of labor, Ezra Gray was born. Their umbilical cord was cut by my partner, and they were placed on my bare chest. The three of us would go on to spend forty-eight more hours in the hospital being monitored and checked for infection. We eventually made it home, and I found myself in the arms of my partner as we wept in the kitchen. We knew that our journey was incredibly taxing, but it cemented our love and commitment to one another. Over the next few days, we would slowly crawl back from the dehydration, sickness, surgery, and overwhelm and find ourselves parents.

Ultimately, this is a blip in the story of my life, but getting pregnant and birthing a child will always be a reminder of the way my body and soul transformed. Though I dreamed of a pregnancy and birth that was smooth, and soft, and gentle, I got something so much more. The struggle was a catalyst for a transformation I never could have imagined. And I cannot think of anything more queer than that.

Halo Dawn

Birthing the World Dragon

"I've got writing work to do today, so Leo will be your grown-up," I tell Ember, who is nearly five. "I'm writing about being pregnant—with you!"

"Can you read it to me?" asks Ember, delighted to be the star of the story.

"Maybe . . ."

"Will it have *sexy things* in it?" they demand gleefully. "Is that why you might not read it to me?"

"I don't know," I reply. "I'll let you know after I've written it."

Why did I want a baby? I always knew I did: I talked about it with two different male partners in my twenties and later asked a female friend if she wanted to co-parent with me (she said no). I promised myself that if I hadn't found a suitable partner by the time I was thirty-five, I'd do it solo. Leo showed up just in time. Our early conversations doubled as co-parent auditions: *How gentle and clear is your communication? How well do you know yourself? How easy it is doing hard things with you?* Very, it turned out. The last eight years have affirmed Team Us as the right choice again and again.

When asked why I wanted to become a parent, I'd say something glib, like: "I'm just competitive—if I see parents disrespecting their kids, I want to prove I can do better. I've got love to give, and I'm excited to help someone discover the world. But mostly because I *really* like snuggles."

I was laughing at myself, but I was also laughing at the question. If I were a cis woman, would anyone ask me why I wanted a baby? Does being queer and trans make my choice to parent so surprising?

I chose another non-binary person as my co-parent. We have queer and trans parent friends now, but at the time I had no role models for trans parenthood.

What was it like being trans and pregnant? Mostly it was like being pregnant. My body spoke to me in body language, a stream of sensory input beyond words. But in the sphere of social interaction, I was misgendered at every turn.

I was assumed to be a woman at prenatal appointments, by midwives, and in every pregnancy book. Pregnancy yoga and baby classes were dominated by women—no other trans people, and almost no dads. I got sick of being called "Mum" by medical professionals, even with my pronouns (they/them) right there at the top of my notes.

In an effort to stem the firehose of cisnormativity, I changed my name by deed poll. I found a trans-friendly doula to advocate for me during labour. I put my new legal name, my pronouns, and my preferred language in my birth plan and smiled encouragingly as midwives hesitated, avoided pronouns altogether, and used my name instead. At least they were trying.

I was more preoccupied with my internal sensations. What pronouns you use makes no difference to the feeling of my ribcage being stretched open from the inside out. It fucking hurts either way.

We announced my pregnancy at a Yule party. During the evening, I quipped to a queer friend, "It's so funny when cis men who fancy me think they're straight. Surprise! You're queer!" It got a laugh—but later one such straight cis man who'd overheard messaged me to mansplain his boner in thirty unsolicited paragraphs of bioessentialism. He cited Judith Butler to dismiss gender as a "performance" irrelevant to his dick, which unerringly twitches in response to procreative partners. There are only two sexes, and only one can get pregnant; this makes me a "mumma" regardless of what I call myself.

Whoa there, tiger! Do I detect the telltale whiff of internalised biphobia? I'd have welcomed feedback critiquing my joke—but I don't appreciate cis people trying to prove my gender wrong.

Butler had that week spoken up against transphobic gender ideology, quoting Simone de Beauvoir: "One is not born a woman but becomes one" (*The Second Sex*, 1949). Butler described how our sex assigned at birth creates a historical context for our developing gender identity: "Nothing about being assigned female at birth determines what kind of life a woman will lead. . . . Indeed, many trans people are assigned one sex at birth, only to claim another one in the course of their lives."[1] Sex and gender are ascribed and produced in an ongoing dialogue between biological and cultural frameworks. Against this backdrop, we are free to relate to our social gender however we wish, and to exert agency upon our sexed bodies.

Splitting a complex system such as sex attributes into two clusters is a choice, and it's only scientifically useful in some circumstances. From hormone insensitivity to natural physiological variation, human sexual characteristics are less a binary than a cloud of attributes which can be grouped in multiple ways.[2]

When I asked him how important chromosomes, hormones, and gamete production actually are to his sexual attraction, my dude replied that he didn't know because his boner had "never been wrong." Call the pope! It's a miracle: a magic dick that always speaks the truth.

Struggling with morning sickness, the last thing I wanted was to defend my gender. Being pregnant made me uniquely sensitive to the ways embodiment intersects with gender expression, identity, and how we're perceived. It's hard to disambiguate the shared experiences of pregnancy from the gendered social expectations that weigh them down—but that doesn't mean we shouldn't try.

> *Is there something inherently queer about pregnancy itself, insofar as it profoundly alters one's "normal" state, and occasions a radical intimacy with—and radical alienation from—one's body? How can an experience so profoundly strange and wild and transformative also symbolize or enact the ultimate conformity?*
>
> —Maggie Nelson, *The Argonauts*

I felt no more or less trans when my nipples got bigger and more sensitive, only curiosity: Bodies are *fascinating*! Growing the machinery to breastfeed was erotically interesting, but mammaries don't feel gendered to me. May every queer who wants them have them and enjoy them! I only really feel dysphoric when people treat me as a woman.

My pregnant body was a trans body, but more to the point it was a chronically ill body; a body with hypothyroidism and polycystic ovary syndrome (PCOS). This was not diagnosed when I was fourteen despite clear signs: severe acne, irregular periods, and blood tests showing "unusually high" testosterone levels. Instead, I was prescribed hormonal contraception to regulate my hormones to cisnormative levels. Disorders of the ovaries and uterus are persistently underdiagnosed, and chronic pain is often dismissed in people treated as women—especially fat people and people of colour.

After living with undiagnosed chronic illness for decades, I told my doctor that I was trying to conceive but not menstruating. Suddenly there were tests and scans in abundance. Even after the diagnosis, I was given no advice about how to manage the condition, only a referral to the fertility clinic. Who cares about quality of life, amiright?! The only help *lady* bodies need is with making babies.

After months of fatigue, I finally learned from friends that PCOS makes me insulin resistant—unable to reliably extract glucose from my blood. A diet high in sugars and quick carbs leaves me disabled by fatigue, brain fog, and chronic inflammation that leads to migraines and painful joints. I changed my diet, saw an immediate reduction in symptoms, and soon afterwards conceived.

I struggled for years without this essential information about my body. That I'm trans makes this a microaggression layer cake, but misogyny sucks for everyone who experiences it. PCOS made far more difference to my experience of pregnancy than being trans did, and being trans did nothing to protect me from institutionalised misogyny.

We were lucky, I know, to be in a trans4trans relationship equipped with the right parts to DIY our conception. We just had to keep putting Tab A into Slot B. Even so, as the months dragged on, Maggie Nelson's poignant line from *The Argonauts* echoed in my head: *What if we called and no baby spirit came.*

"It's only taking so long because we keep forgetting to have PIV," I joked. "Why can't we get pregnant from stimulating Leo's prostate?"

After prioritising baby-growing for years, I can now finally centre myself in how I care for my body. I started low-dose testosterone when Ember was four. I still need to watch my diet and take my thyroid meds, but testosterone makes me feel vigorous, full of vitality. With every increase in muscle, energy, and clit growth, I feel more at home in myself. I'm tickled to shave the whiskers on my chin, as patchy as any teen boy. I wasn't conscious of dysphoria before, but I'm definitely feeling euphoria now.

We put great stock in hormones. When I started hormone therapy, the PCOS symptoms seemed to go away overnight. Does my trans body "naturally" need more testosterone than it makes by itself, or had the stress of putting my baby's needs before my own been taking a greater toll than I'd realised? Perhaps it was just coincidence; a new era of taking better care of myself in multiple ways. As with a child, caring for my body is a mystery, a complex system I can't fully comprehend. All I can do is try things and see what works.

I was pregnant for two months before I realised. When debilitating fatigue struck again in the autumn, I chalked it up to PCOS. It wasn't until I was kept up one night by severe pelvic pain that I went to the doctor—who told me I was pregnant. And the pain? Sometimes it "just happens."

I finally noticed the swelling and tenderness in my breasts. Two weeks earlier during a breast bondage scene, I'd actually started lactating. I remember saying with perfect innocence: "Wow, bodies are amazing—I'm not even pregnant!"

Bodies *are* amazing, but they also suck. My first trimester was wiped out by nausea. So much for the PCOS diet—all I could keep down was fruit and crackers. I didn't want to tell friends until we got the certainty of the twelve-week scan, but the isolation was miserable.

The worst day was going to get my new tattoo finished, which I'd been looking forward to for weeks. I mentioned my pregnancy in passing, thinking I might need to take a break to manage nausea. "Oh," she said, "I can't work on you, we're not insured. We can't take the risk."

"What risk?"

"Well, if you get blood poisoning, it might harm the baby."

Never mind that I'd been fine every previous tattoo session, that I was willing to sign a waiver. I was carrying a foetus, so my body was no longer my own. This tattoo was a celebration of my curves, a gift for myself after the long and uncomfortable journey this body had been on—but I wasn't allowed it. I started ugly crying before I'd even left the studio. It all landed on me at once: the infantilisation, the helplessness, the paternalistic bullshit that treats pregnant people as walking incubators. I got lucky that our second trimester holiday was scheduled just before the twenty-eight-week cutoff—beyond that point, I'd have needed a doctor's note to be allowed to fly. If the timing had been slightly different, I'd have been turned away at the airport. I dreaded every choice taken away from me because of my pregnancy, but I never saw them coming.

In early January, after the twelve-week scan gave us the all-clear, we made a public announcement. Leo's work involves fabrication and 3D printing, so I found a foetus model on Thingiverse and we printed it and posted a photo of us holding it with the legend "HUMAN 3D PRINTING IN PROGRESS, ESTIMATED DATE OF DELIVERY JULY 2019."

In the second trimester, I claimed as much freedom as I could. I bleached my hair and dyed it pink, then got it cut into a short style with shaved sides at the local barbers. I faithfully attended tai chi twice a week—I wanted to get as fit as possible before the birth. I also went to a rave festival, where I stayed sober, ate three meals a day, stubbornly ignored my acid reflux, and danced to my heart's content. I went to another music festival and a Burning Man regional gathering before the baby was born, along with a film festival and a five-day professional development course. I knew it was my last chance to have these experiences without parenting responsibilities for a while. The baby was very wriggly, sometimes delivering Super Rolling Attack Combos into my internal organs for over a quarter of an hour, but they always settled down when I got onto the dance floor. Come to think of it, they do still like fat bass lines.

At the twenty-week scan, we were firm about not wanting to know the assumed sex of the baby. We researched gender-neutral names and found several we liked. Parent friends donated us baby clothes; we arrived at one house to find a mum-to-be just leaving. "She's having a boy, so I'm afraid she's rinsed the blue ones," our friend apologised. We were left with everything deemed "girly": pink and white and frills and bunnies. We dyed them all purple.

Meanwhile, my boobs were getting bigger. I'd always avoided bras: They gave me backache, and they made me dysphoric. But I couldn't put it off any longer. I found sleep nursing bras with soft bands and crossover cups in jersey cotton. Once I was spurting milk everywhere,

I was grateful to have somewhere to tuck the cotton pads. Wearing a bra was weird, but I also enjoyed the transformation. With a shaved head and giant milk squirters sticking out whichever way I turned, I felt like Tank Girl.

In *Trans Like Me*, CN Lester describes gender dysphoria as a mismatch in proprioception: "like missing a step in the dark, when you're convinced that the step is actually there until the moment you hit the ground."[3] Pregnancy was a lot like that: My proprioception never did catch up with my bump. I kept scraping it on door handles and furniture corners. I think it was easier to enjoy the changes because I knew they were temporary, but there are ways in which I'm still not used to my post-baby body.

Gender transition and pregnancy are physical transformations which offer opportunities for autonomy and surrender. I chose to get pregnant, just as I'm now choosing to take testosterone, but in neither case can I predict how exactly it will affect my body. Trans people and pregnant people alike have to deal with medical gatekeeping and paternalistic legislation denying our bodily autonomy. After my consensual pregnancy, my pro-choice politics are rock solid: No-one should ever do this who doesn't want to.

In the second trimester, Leo and I went to an exhibition called *Oxytocin* featuring art by "mothers" about "motherhood." What most stayed with me was a series of huge black-and-white self-portrait photographs of a mother lying catatonic, staring blankly into space in a squalid apartment, two children frolicking gleefully amongst the mess. Her kids must have had a blast helping her shoot them. In the months following Ember's birth, I often thought about the listlessness and emptiness she embodies in those photos. It was validating to know I wasn't alone as I felt the same exhaustion drag on me during the long, isolated days of pandemic parenting. Parents need space to talk about these feelings, especially given the uncelebrated nature of childcare. But we aren't all mothers.

On the panel discussion, I heard Del LaGrace Volcano, a genderqueer, intersex artist and activist, speak about their queer, gender-creative family and using tubes to nipple-feed their firstborn from a bottle of milk expressed by their partner. I wanted Leo to take hormones and induce lactation so we could share the labour and experience of breastfeeding. There were new articles about trans women successfully breastfeeding their children,[4] and in 2002 Agence France-Presse reported on a Sri Lankan father who nursed his two daughters after his wife died in childbirth. Bodies are magic!

I know Leo has at times felt dysphoric about their flat chest, but ultimately they didn't feel sufficiently well resourced to try to nurse Ember. During my pregnancy, Leo was struggling with mobility issues and chronic pain while waiting for a hip replacement. How would hormones affect the delicate balance of their vitality? We couldn't access gender-affirming care for transfeminine lactation, not on the timescale we needed, and Leo didn't want to risk DIY hormone therapy without medical supervision. If we'd had access to trans-friendly health care and could have seen a consultant, that door might have opened; going through it would have changed the whole balance of our lives during Ember's babyhood.

I got over my disappointment and embraced my role as "boob parent"—I even chose the parent nickname "Boo" for short. I enjoyed the close cuddles and the powerful feeling of creating food from my body. I became Ember's sleep aid, and their source of comfort and nourishment. When they needed me, I had to drop everything and go. For twenty months, we couldn't spend a night apart, and they nursed regularly until they were two years old. As the more able-bodied parent, I wore them constantly in the sling and did most of the domestic work before and after Leo's surgery, my body getting stronger, my shoulders more hench. Carrying the baby, all our bags, and pushing Leo's wheelchair to the park, I felt like Power Dad. But when I hung washing on the line and dug earth for planting with Ember wrapped on my back, I felt connected to a lineage of birth-givers and baby-wearers spanning thousands of generations.

By the time Ember's teeth came through and they kept biting me during night feeds, I was done. But weaning was slow, and it was over a year before I could tolerate erotic nipple touch again. I've stayed up late researching options for non-flat top surgery, looking into breast reduction (and sometimes enlargement—what can I say, my gender is fluid). But now that my nipples are my own again, I don't want to risk losing sensation.

I'm forty this year, and I have the body of someone who's given birth. Saggy breasts and a fat tummy are less conventionally attractive, but fuck convention. The small, perky boobs I had when I was twenty would look wrong on this body. I fed my child from these tits; they're a proud part of my story.

A few weeks after starting testosterone, I dreamed that I looked in the mirror and saw a scrawny goblin boy looking back, flat-chested, his ears sticking out like my uncle's—and felt intensely dysphoric. I woke up feeling relieved to have clarity. The boobs stay, testosterone-reduced and all. I feel as euphoric disguising them under a waistcoat as I do dangling them in my lover's face.

I researched options and wrote my birth plan: a home birth with a birth pool, no induction, no unnecessary interventions, optimal cord clamping, no assigning a gender to the baby. The birth books were all by women, for women. Being a trans parent feels like being a baleen whale, taking in masses of information, digesting the bits worth keeping, and letting my filtering system spit all the cisnormative crap back out.

When I read Elizabeth Davis and Debra Pascali-Bonaro say in *Orgasmic Birth* that pregnant "women" need close women confidantes because male partners can't provide emotional support, I nearly spat out my tea. Men, you see, have their language centre on one side of their brain and their emotions on the other, making them neurologically incapable of talking about feelings. He can't help it—he's just cognitively challenged!

I threw the book across the room, but I didn't want to throw the baby out with the bathwater. The idea of riding the waves of strong sensation as if birth were the most intense tantric sex of my life remained compelling. In the third trimester, Leo and I enjoyed perineal massage and "stretchy" sex. Encompassing their whole hand put me one step closer to stretching around a baby's head, right?

During the latent phase of labour, we did our best to get the oxytocin flowing. Our doula stepped out of the room, and I sat on Leo's lap while we made out and they stroked my nipples. The pleasure certainly made the contractions more intense. But when I entered the active phase, there was no time for such dalliances—and no need. I was buffeted by nonstop, agonising contractions, each one a fist squeezing the middle of my body to a pulp.

I laboured at home for twenty-seven hours before transferring to the birth centre, because my waters hadn't broken. There was a pool there too, but they wouldn't let Leo be naked—although the home birth team hadn't batted an eyelid. Now we were on their turf; the medical establishment had categorised Leo as a "man," and their body therefore unacceptable. I would have been more furious about it if I hadn't been busy giving birth.

I will never forget the sensation of my pelvic bones moving apart to make way for Ember's descent through my body: the intense pressure, the momentous feeling of being broken open. I felt the contours of their face pressing and moving against my sensitive inner walls. It was like being fisted by a giant. Gravity eased the head lower as I breathed through each contraction, stretching my patience and my membranes to their limits. I remember the incredible, crushing pressure against my urethra and clitoris, the burning sensation in my perineum. Why hadn't anyone offered me lube? And then the body being born in a great, slippery rush; the exquisite feeling of my baby's soft, creamy limbs slipping out of me. Was it orgasmic? No. But it was an extraordinary release, a peak experience.

I gathered them up and leaned back into Leo's arms. *Hello,* I thought, *who are you?* This little stranger had come into our lives, a small, unfamiliar body. A whole new person.

Childbirth was a rite of passage. No matter how nerdy your research, nothing can truly prepare you. I have an immense respect for everyone who has done it, regardless of the details. It blows my mind that every human who has ever existed was brought into the world by someone labouring, enduring, and somehow birthing a baby. Each of us is the result of an unbroken chain of our ancestors successfully giving birth, mostly without pain relief or medical care, going back three hundred thousand years. It's an ancient, sacred heritage. I feel honoured to be part of it—not as a woman (many women never get pregnant or give birth, after all), but in a way that transcends gender.

Alex Iantaffi talks in their podcast *Gender Stories* about gender liberation in the context of healing justice: the work of healing the effects of trauma and oppression on our bodies, minds, and hearts. After millennia of uterus owners having little reproductive autonomy and being treated as an oppressed class, healing is sorely needed. That means decolonising our ideas about bodies and gender and advocating for bodily autonomy for all humans.

Pregnancy and parenthood connect me with a global community of birth-givers and care-givers: mums, dads, and every queer, trans, and non-binary person who has borne or raised a child. Throughout most of history, I would have been treated as a woman; expanding my gender beyond "woman" is part of imagining a more expansive future for all of us.

> *I don't feel any less of a woman now; I just know there are so many other parts of me that are now welcome because I've let go of that identity.*
>
> —Z Griss, "Living in Attunement with Sensation Rather than Identity," *Queer Magic*

I go downstairs to make tea and find Leo and Ember in the dining room. "I created the world and everything in it," Ember is saying. "I'm a dragon and I created the whole of planet Earth!"

I get out my gel packet and apply testosterone to my upper arms, smoothing my palms over increasingly rounded muscles and the darker hairs that are starting to appear. When Ember tries to climb on me, I give them their daily reminder that I need to wash my hands before I can hug them.

"How does it feel to have incarnated the World Dragon?" Leo asks.

I smile. "Humbling."

Notes

1 Judith Butler, "The Backlash Against 'Gender Ideology' Must Stop," *New Statesman*, January 21, 2019, https://www.newstatesman.com/culture/2019/01/judith-butler-backlash-against-gender-ideology-must-stop.

2 ScienceVet (@ScienceVet2), "Biological sex is a spectrum," Twitter (now X), August 30, 2018, https://x.com/ScienceVet2/status/1035246030500061184.

3 CN Lester, *Trans Like Me: Conversations for All of Us* (Seal Press, 2018).

4 Tamar Reisman and Zil Goldstein, "Case Report: Induced Lactation in a Transgender Woman," *Transgender Health* 3, no. 1 (2018): 24–26, http://dx.doi.org/10.1089/trgh.2017.0044.

Acknowledgments

I thank my parents, Jan and Martin. I am blessed to return to them again and again—my father here, and my mother in spirit and memory. With each turn on life's journey, I find a new facet of their humanity and wisdom. I thank my sister, Emily, whose encouragement pushed this into reality and who has been a supporter and thought partner in all my endeavors. I thank my wonderful family members Eric, Annika, and Cleo. I thank Adriel, Andrew, Bakari, Catherine, Charles, Darcy, Edith, Jeff, Jon, Judi, Kamilah, Kelly, marissa, Melissa, Milvia, Rebecca, Regula, Steven, Tomas, and Wade. I thank my extended family, my friends, and my teachers. I thank Kayla Eckard for her excellent editorial support. I thank all the contributors, and the friends, colleagues, and writing groups who supported us in bringing our stories to the page. I thank my ancestors and all those who came before me in movements large and small. I thank those who come after me, who inspire and motivate me. I thank the Duwamish people: past, present, and future stewards of the (unceded) beautiful place I call home. I especially thank O and Y, my beloved, brilliant, cherished children.

About the Contributors

Felix Aster (he/him) is a California-based writer and parent of settler descent. He is interested in relational, collective, and land-based trauma stewardship.

Amari Ayomide (they/them) is a Black, trans + queer activist, community leader, and storyteller. They are a certified Peer Support Counselor in the state of Washington and currently work as Black Led Organizing & Initiatives Coordinator with Queer the Land. They center their work on restorative practices centering disability justice + care, and they share their story with the empowerment of their community in mind.

Jacoby Ballard (he/him) is a social justice educator and yoga teacher. With twenty-five years of experience at the nexus of liberation and embodiment, he leads workshops, retreats, and segments in teacher trainings, presents at conferences, and has been an artist-in-residence on dozens of college campuses. Jacoby has taught in schools, hospitals, nonprofit and business offices, a maximum security prison, a recovery center, a cancer center, LGBT centers, gyms, a veterans' center, and yoga studios. He is a cofounder of Third Root Community Health Center, which operated in Brooklyn for thirteen years, currently serves on the board of the Buddhist Peace Fellowship, and is the author of *A Queer Dharma: Yoga and Meditations for Liberation.*

Jamie Cayley (he/they), originally from Guatemala, lived and studied in the UK before moving to the US to pursue a graduate degree at the Brown School at Washington University in St. Louis. He loved

Orla Gartland, Cavetown, and his cat, Willow. He cared very deeply for his friends and his community and volunteered with St. Louis Queer Support & Healing (SQSH), Trans Lifeline, and the Trevor Project. He had a passion for queer youth outreach and mental health support. Jamie was a soft-spoken and gentle presence, and he is cherished and missed. A portion of the proceeds from this book will go to SQSH in his memory.

Halo Dawn (they/them) is a parent, writer, and activist living in Bristol. They are the author of "Gender-Creative Parenting and Me" in the anthology *Gender Euphoria: Stories of Joy from Trans, Non-Binary and Intersex Writers.* Their passions currently include wild swimming, Brazilian jiu-jitsu, somatic psychology and embodied approaches to healing, and self-directed learning for people of all ages.

Lífthrasir Green (he/him) is an artist, parent, and advocate for the right to abortion and bodily autonomy. After writing his essay, Lífthrasir learned about Ursula K. Le Guin's essay (and video) "What It Was Like" from the book *Words Are My Matter.* He dedicates his essay to her, as well as everyone who has had an abortion and everyone who has worked to make abortion safe and legal.

J.F. Gutfreund (they/them) is a white non-binary trans midwife born and raised in Cincinnati, Ohio. Their life work has emerged at the intersections of reproductive justice, healing work, and antiracism practice. They live in Tiwa and Tewa country and have been influenced and mentored immeasurably by the communities of northern New Mexico, offering them a place to learn, collaborate, and grow over the past eighteen years. They are raising two children with a beloved community, practicing their liberation politics through the relentless joy and exhaustion of parenting.

Amber Hickey (they/them) is an assistant professor of art history. Amber's writing most often explores the intersections of activism, art, decolonization, and environmental justice. They live in Chattanooga with their partner and two cute kiddos.

Kara Johnson Martone (they/she) is a therapist, activist, and cofounder of the Liberation Coalition, a collective of trans, queer, and BIPOC mental health professionals in Denver, Colorado. Kara has worked as an advocate for the queer community for over a decade. In 2023, Kara was a recipient of the Denver Business Journal DEI Award for work in building business and policies centering queer and marginalized voices.

Dr. S. Aakash Kishore (they/he) is a clinical psychologist and proud gestational parent. They navigate themes of QTBIPOC joy, grief, and ritual in their clinical practice, daily life, and written work.

Simon Knaphus (he/him) is a trans dad and Social Security disability attorney. His publications include essays in *Rad Dad: Dispatches from the Frontiers of Fatherhood* and *Rad Families: A Celebration*. Simon also consulted for the *Lunasea Scout Guide for Breastfeeding Families* and *Harm Reduction Hacks*. He is a 2025 Seattle Public Library Writers' Room Resident.

Dr. Simone Kolysh (they/them) is a sociologist and a life coach at Defiant Life Coaching. They hold degrees in biology, public health, and sociology and wrote *Everyday Violence: The Public Harassment of Women and LGBTQ People*. They teach women's studies part-time and coach neurodivergent, LGBTQ, and marginalized people the rest of the time.

Zillah Rose (they/them) likes to accumulate skills that can assist them as a fae-witch, garden witch, and kitchen witch. They aspire to write more often, fully grow their own medicinal plant garden, make more baked goods from wild roses and nettles, and continue to learn American Sign Language with their kiddo. They also enjoy playing strategy board games in their minimal spare time.

Kathy Slaughter (they/them) loves watching people bloom as they move through painful life lessons and find belonging. In addition to impacting hundreds of psychotherapy clients, their accomplishments include a TEDx Talk titled "Love Lessons from Open Relationships" and hosting the conference "The Practices and Principles of Ethical Polyamory." They live in Indiana with their partners and new baby.

g k somers (they/them) is a transgender non-binary solo parent by choice and is thrilled to make their writing debut as a part of this anthology representing seahorse parents. somers is primarily a facilitator and educator working in the nonprofit arts industry and currently works with students and educators on issues of equity and transformative representation. in their spare time, somers can be found adventuring with their toddler, convening community, playing music, and dreaming up new possibilities.

Tom (they/them) is a Seattle-based creative soul finding their way through life by hand building with clay, parenting with heart, thoughtful community building, and digging around in the dirt—occasionally enabling something to grow.

Sam Vanbelle (they/them) is an illustrator based in Antwerp, Belgium. They make playful, easy, readable, and well-thought-out images. They draw for a wide range of clients: brands, publishing houses, nonprofit organizations, magazines, newspapers, and more. They have a keen eye for diversity and representation in their illustrations. Sam teaches illustration at Sint Lucas Antwerpen. As part of Sint Lucas Antwerp Research Group, they work around gender, binaries, and illustration. At home, they are happy to spend their days with their girlfriend, Tessa, and their kid, Bruna. They're proud of their trans pregnancy and their queer family.

J. Workman (they/them) is a civil rights attorney and writer based in Kerhonkson, New York. They are white, queer, and transmasc. Aside from a piece in a social work textbook, this is J's first publication. These days you might find them reading about forest farming, trying to speak up more, trading jokes with their three-year-old, or riding the mighty waves of early middle age.

ABOUT PM PRESS

PM Press is an independent, radical publisher of critically necessary books for our tumultuous times. Our aim is to deliver bold political ideas and vital stories to all walks of life and arm the dreamers to demand the impossible. Founded in 2007 by a small group of people with decades of publishing, media, and organizing experience, we have sold millions of copies of our books, most often one at a time, face to face. We're old enough to know what we're doing and young enough to know what's at stake. Join us to create a better world.

PM Press
PO Box 23912
Oakland, CA 94623
www.pmpress.org

PM Press in Europe
europe@pmpress.org
www.pmpress.org.uk

FRIENDS OF PM PRESS

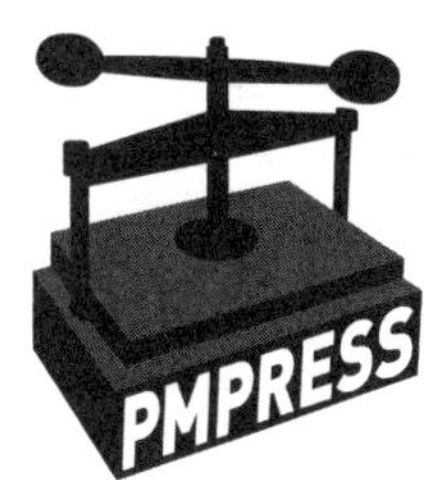

These are indisputably momentous times—the financial system is melting down globally and the Empire is stumbling. Now more than ever there is a vital need for radical ideas.

In the many years since its founding—and on a mere shoestring—PM Press has risen to the formidable challenge of publishing and distributing knowledge and entertainment for the struggles ahead. With hundreds of releases to date, we have published an impressive and stimulating array of literature, art, music, politics, and culture. Using every available medium, we've succeeded in connecting those hungry for ideas and information to those putting them into practice.

Friends of PM allows you to directly help impact, amplify, and revitalize the discourse and actions of radical writers, filmmakers, and artists. It provides us with a stable foundation from which we can build upon our early successes and provides a much-needed subsidy for the materials that can't necessarily pay their own way. You can help make that happen—and receive every new title automatically delivered to your door once a month—by joining as a Friend of PM Press. And, we'll throw in a free T-shirt when you sign up.

Here are your options:

- **$30 a month** Get all books and pamphlets plus a 50% discount on all webstore purchases
- **$40 a month** Get all PM Press releases (including CDs and DVDs) plus a 50% discount on all webstore purchases
- **$100 a month** Superstar—Everything plus PM merchandise, free downloads, and a 50% discount on all webstore purchases

For those who can't afford $30 or more a month, we have **Sustainer Rates** at $15, $10, and $5. Sustainers get a free PM Press T-shirt and a 50% discount on all purchases from our website.

Your Visa or Mastercard will be billed once a month, until you tell us to stop. Or until our efforts succeed in bringing the revolution around. Or the financial meltdown of Capital makes plastic redundant. Whichever comes first.

Revolutionary Mothering: Love on the Front Lines

Edited by Alexis Pauline Gumbs, China Martens, and Mai'a Williams with a Preface by Loretta J. Ross

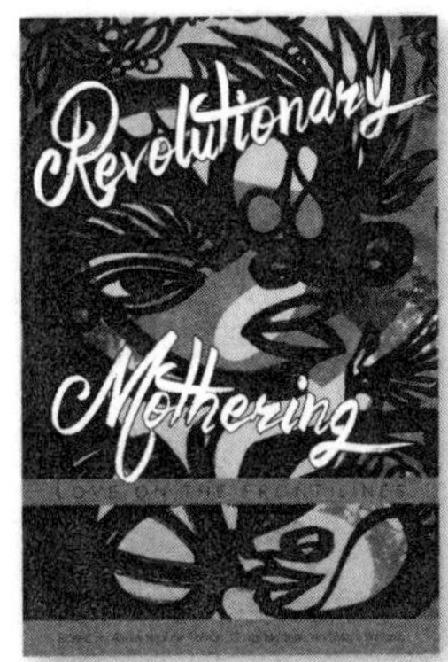

ISBN: 978-1-62963-110-3
$17.95 272 pages

Inspired by the legacy of radical and queer black feminists of the 1970s and '80s, *Revolutionary Mothering* places marginalized mothers of color at the center of a world of necessary transformation. The challenges we face as movements working for racial, economic, reproductive, gender, and food justice, as well as anti-violence, anti-imperialist, and queer liberation, are the same challenges that many mothers face every day. Oppressed mothers create a generous space for life in the face of life-threatening limits, activate a powerful vision of the future while navigating tangible concerns in the present, move beyond individual narratives of choice toward collective solutions, live for more than ourselves, and remain accountable to a future that we cannot always see. *Revolutionary Mothering* is a movement-shifting anthology committed to birthing new worlds, full of faith and hope for what we can raise up together.

Contributors include June Jordan, Malkia A. Cyril, Esteli Juarez, Cynthia Dewi Oka, Fabiola Sandoval, Sumayyah Talibah, Victoria Law, Tara Villalba, Lola Mondragón, Christy NaMee Eriksen, Norma Angelica Marrun, Vivian Chin, Rachel Broadwater, Autumn Brown, Layne Russell, Noemi Martinez, Katie Kaput, alba onofrio, Gabriela Sandoval, Cheryl Boyce Taylor, Ariel Gore, Claire Barrera, Lisa Factora-Borchers, Fabielle Georges, H. Bindy K. Kang, Terri Nilliasca, Irene Lara, Panquetzani, Mamas of Color Rising, tk karakashian tunchez, Arielle Julia Brown, Lindsey Campbell, Micaela Cadena, and Karen Su.

"This collection is a treat for anyone that sees class and that needs to learn more about the experiences of women of color (and who doesn't?!). There is no dogma here, just fresh ideas and women of color taking on capitalism, anti-racist, anti-sexist theory-building that is rooted in the most primal of human connections, the making of two people from the body of one: mothering."
—Barbara Jensen, author of *Reading Classes: On Culture and Classism in America*

"For women of color, mothering—the art of mothering—has been framed by the most virulent systems, historically: enslavement, colonialism, capitalism, imperialism. We have had few opportunities to define mothering not only as an aspect of individual lives and choices, but as the processes of love and as a way of structuring community. Revolutionary Mothering *arrives as a needed balm."*
—Alexis De Veaux, author of *Warrior Poet: A Biography of Audre Lorde*

Rad Families: A Celebration

Edited by Tomas Moniz
with a Foreword by Ariel Gore

ISBN: 978-1-62963-230-8
$19.95 296 pages

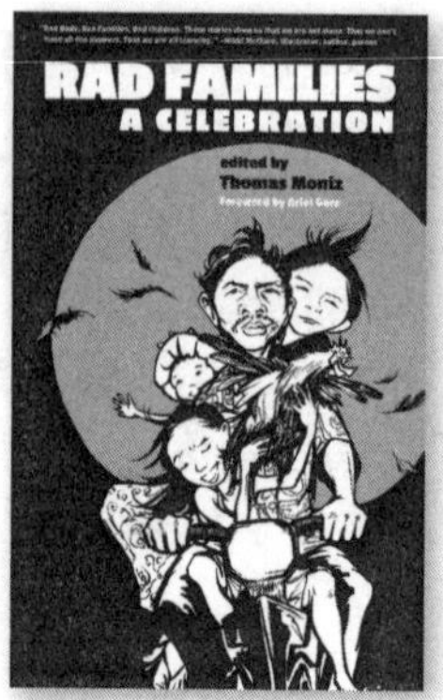

Rad Families: A Celebration honors the messy, the painful, the playful, the beautiful, the myriad ways we create families. This is not an anthology of experts, or how-to articles on perfect parenting; it often doesn't even try to provide answers. Instead, the writers strive to be honest and vulnerable in sharing their stories and experiences, their failures and their regrets.

Gathering parents and writers from diverse communities, it explores the process of getting pregnant from trans birth to adoption, grapples with issues of racism and police brutality, probes raising feminists and feminist parenting. It plumbs the depths of empty nesting and letting go.

Some contributors are recognizable authors and activists but most are everyday parents working and loving and trying to build a better world one diaper change at a time. It's a book that reminds us all that we are not alone, that community can help us get through the difficulties, can, in fact, make us better people. It's a celebration, join us!

Contributors include Jonas Cannon, Ian MacKaye, Burke Stansbury, Danny Goot, Simon Knaphus, Artnoose, Welch Canavan, Daniel Muro LaMere, Jennifer Lewis, Zach Ellis, Alicia Dornadic, Jesse Palmer, Mindi J., Carla Bergman, Tasnim Nathoo, Rachel Galindo, Robert Liu-Trujillo, Dawn Caprice, Shawn Taylor, D.A. Begay, Philana Dollin, Airial Clark, Allison Wolfe, Roger Porter, cubbie rowland-storm, Annakai & Rob Geshlider, Jeremy Adam Smith, Frances Hardinge, Jonathan Shipley, Bronwyn Davies Glover, Amy Abugo Ongiri, Mike Araujo, Craig Elliott, Eleanor Wohlfeiler, Scott Hoshida, Plinio Hernandez, Madison Young, Nathan Torp, Sasha Vodnik, Jessie Susannah, Krista Lee Hanson, Carvell Wallace, Dani Burlison, Brian Whitman, scott winn, Kermit Playfoot, Chris Crass, and Zora Moniz.

"Rad dads, rad families, rad children. These stories show us that we are not alone. That we don't have all the answers. That we are all learning."
—Nikki McClure, illustrator, author, parent

"Rad Families *is the collection for all families."*
—Innosanto Nagara, author/illustrator of *A Is for Activist*

Rad Dad: Dispatches from the Frontiers of Fatherhood

Edited by Jeremy Adam Smith and Tomas Moniz

ISBN: 978-1-60486-481-6
$15.00 200 pages

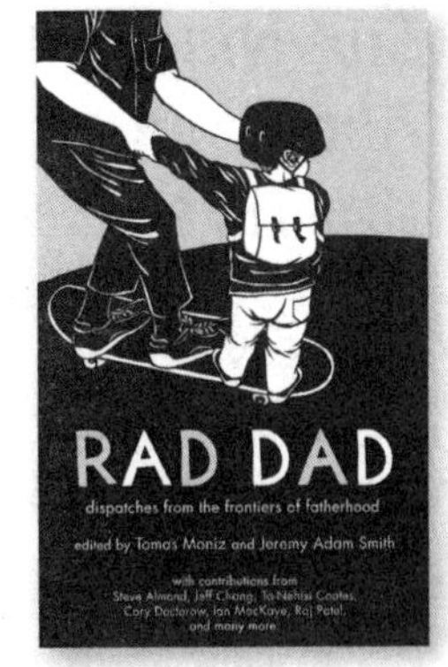

Rad Dad: Dispatches from the Frontiers of Fatherhood combines the best pieces from the award-winning zine *Rad Dad* and from the blog Daddy Dialectic, two kindred publications that have tried to explore parenting as political territory. Both of these projects have pushed the conversation around fathering beyond the safe, apolitical focus most books and websites stick to; they have not been complacent but have worked hard to create a diverse, multi-faceted space in which to grapple with the complexity of fathering. Today more than ever, fatherhood demands constant improvisation, risk, and struggle. With grace and honesty and strength, *Rad Dad*'s writers tackle all the issues that other parenting guides are afraid to touch: the brutalities, beauties, and politics of the birth experience, the challenges of parenting on an equal basis with mothers, the tests faced by transgendered and gay fathers, the emotions of sperm donation, and parental confrontations with war, violence, racism, and incarceration. *Rad Dad* is for every father out in the real world trying to parent in ways that are loving, meaningful, authentic, and ultimately revolutionary.

Contributors include: Steve Almond, Jack Amoureux, Mike Araujo, Mark Andersen, Jeff Chang, Ta-Nehisi Coates, Jeff Conant, Sky Cosby, Jason Denzin, Cory Doctorow, Craig Elliott, Chip Gagnon, Keith Hennessy, David L. Hoyt, Simon Knapus, Ian MacKaye, Tomas Moniz, Zappa Montag, Raj Patel, Jeremy Adam Smith, Jason Sperber, Burke Stansbury, Shawn Taylor, Tata, Jeff West, and Mark Whiteley.

"Rad Dad *gives voice to egalitarian parenting and caregiving by men in a truly radical fashion, with its contributors challenging traditional norms of what it means to be a father and subverting paradigms, while making you laugh in the process. With its thoughtful and engaging stories on topics like birth, stepfathering, gender, politics, pop culture, and the challenges of kids growing older, this collection of essays and interviews is a compelling addition to books on fatherhood."*
—Jennifer Silverman, co-editor, *My Baby Rides the Short Bus: The Unabashedly Human Experience of Raising Kids with Disabilities*

Surviving the Future: Abolitionist Queer Strategies

Edited by Scott Branson, Raven Hudson, and Bry Reed with a Foreword by Mimi Thi Nguyen

ISBN: 978-1-62963-971-0
$22.95 328 pages

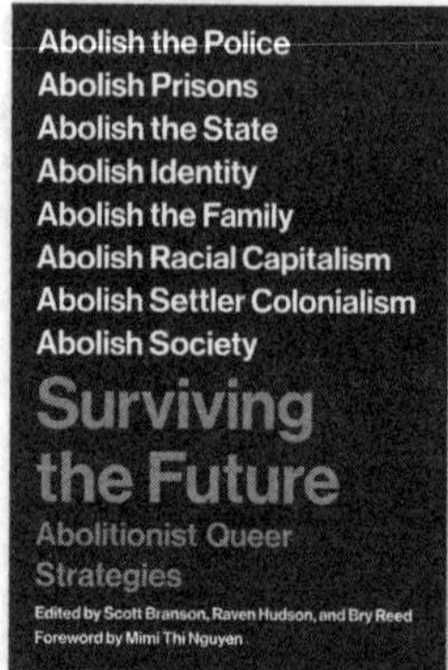

Surviving the Future is a collection of the most current ideas in radical queer movement work and revolutionary queer theory. Beset by a new pandemic, fanning the flames of global uprising, these queers cast off progressive narratives of liberal hope while building mutual networks of rebellion and care. These essays propose a militant strategy of queer survival in an ever-precarious future. Starting from a position of abolition—of prisons, police, the State, identity, and racist cisheteronormative society—this collection refuses the bribes of inclusion in a system built on our expendability. Though the mainstream media saturates us with the boring norms of queer representation (with a recent focus on trans visibility), the writers in this book ditch false hope to imagine collective visions of liberation that tell different stories, build alternate worlds, and refuse the legacies of racial capitalism, anti-Blackness, and settler colonialism. The work curated in this book spans Black queer life in the time of COVID-19 and uprising, assimilation and pinkwashing settler colonial projects, subversive and deviant forms of representation, building anarchist trans/queer infrastructures, and more. Contributors include Che Gossett, Yasmin Nair, Mattilda Bernstein Sycamore, Adrian Shanker, Kitty Stryker, Toshio Meronek, and more.

"Surviving the Future *is a testament that otherwise worlds are not only possible, our people are making them right now—and they are queering how we get there through organizing and intellectual work. Now is the perfect time to interrogate how we are with each other and the land we inhabit. This collection gives us ample room to do just that in a moment of mass uprisings led by everyday people demanding safety without policing, prisons and other forms of punishment.*
—Charlene A. Carruthers, author of *Unapologetic: A Black, Queer, and Feminist Mandate for Radical Movements*

"Surviving the Future *is not an anthology that simply includes queer and trans minorities in mix of existing abolitionist thought. Rather, it is a transformative collection of queer/trans methods for living an abolitionist life. Anyone who dreams of dismantling the prison-industrial complex, policing, borders and the surveillance state should read this book. Frankly, everybody who doesn't share that dream should read it, too, and maybe they'll start dreaming differently."*
—Susan Stryker, author of *Transgender History: The Roots of Today's Revolution*

Birth Work as Care Work: Stories from Activist Birth Communities

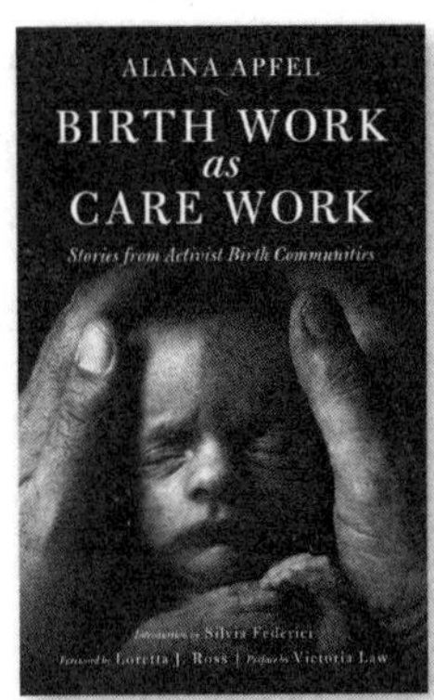

Alana Apfel, with a Foreword by Loretta J. Ross, Preface by Victoria Law, and Introduction by Silvia Federici

ISBN: 978-1-62963-151-6
$14.95 128 pages

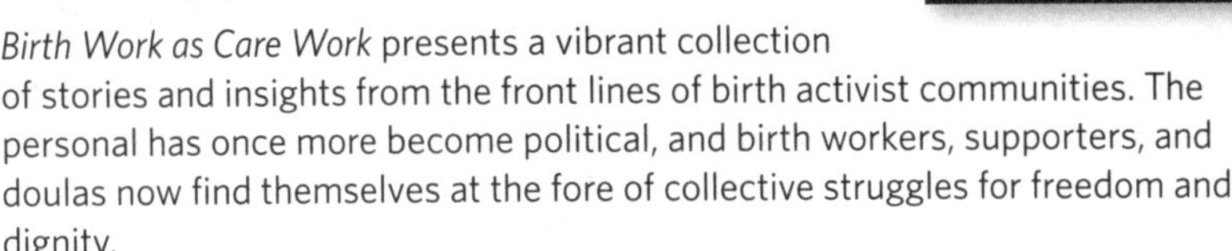

Birth Work as Care Work presents a vibrant collection of stories and insights from the front lines of birth activist communities. The personal has once more become political, and birth workers, supporters, and doulas now find themselves at the fore of collective struggles for freedom and dignity.

The author, herself a scholar and birth justice organizer, provides a unique platform to explore the political dynamics of birth work; drawing connections between birth, reproductive labor, and the struggles of caregiving communities today. Articulating a politics of care work in and through the reproductive process, the book brings diverse voices into conversation to explore multiple possibilities and avenues for change.

At a moment when agency over our childbirth experiences is increasingly centralized in the hands of professional elites, *Birth Work as Care Work* presents creative new ways to reimagine the trajectory of our reproductive processes. Most importantly, the contributors present new ways of thinking about the entire life cycle, providing a unique and creative entry point into the essence of all human struggle—the struggle over the reproduction of life itself.

"I love this book, all of it. The polished essays and the interviews with birth workers dare to take on the deepest questions of human existence."
—Carol Downer, cofounder of the Feminist Women's Health Centers of California and author of *A Woman's Book of Choices*

"This volume provides theoretically rich, practical tools for birth and other care workers to collectively and effectively fight capitalism and the many intersecting processes of oppression that accompany it. Birth Work as Care Work *forcefully and joyfully reminds us that the personal is political, a lesson we need now more than ever."*
—Adrienne Pine, author of *Working Hard, Drinking Hard: On Violence and Survival in Honduras*

Raising Free People: Unschooling as Liberation and Healing Work

Akilah S. Richards
with a Foreword by Bayo Akomolafe

ISBN: 978-1-62963-833-1
$17.00 192 pages

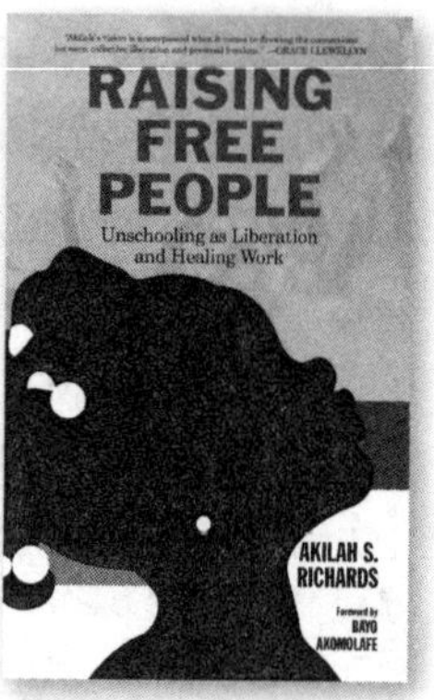

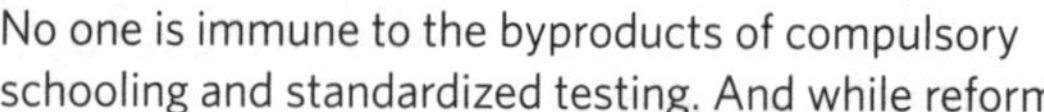
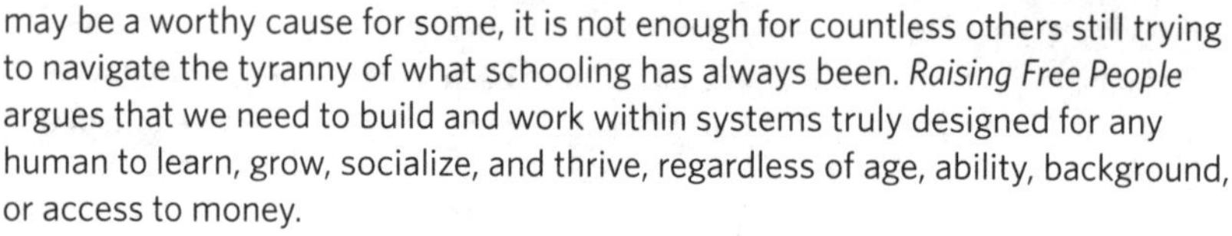
No one is immune to the byproducts of compulsory schooling and standardized testing. And while reform may be a worthy cause for some, it is not enough for countless others still trying to navigate the tyranny of what schooling has always been. *Raising Free People* argues that we need to build and work within systems truly designed for any human to learn, grow, socialize, and thrive, regardless of age, ability, background, or access to money.

Families and conscious organizations across the world are healing generations of school wounds by pivoting into self-directed, intentional community-building, and *Raising Free People* shows you exactly how unschooling can help facilitate this process.

Individual experiences influence our approach to parenting and education, so we need more than the rules, tools, and "bad adult" guilt trips found in so many parenting and education books. We need to reach behind our behaviors to seek and find our triggers; to examine and interrupt the ways that social issues such as colonization still wreak havoc on our ability to trust ourselves, let alone children. *Raising Free People* explores examples of the transition from school or homeschooling to unschooling, how single parents and people facing financial challenges unschool successfully, and the ways unschooling allows us to address generational trauma and unlearn the habits we mindlessly pass on to children.

In these detailed and unabashed stories and insights, Richards examines the ways that her relationships to blackness, decolonization, and healing work all combine to form relationships and enable community-healing strategies rooted in an unschooling practice. This is how millions of families center human connection, practice clear and honest communication, and raise children who do not grow up to feel that they narrowly survived their childhoods.

"This is an insightful, brilliant book by one of today's most inspiring leaders in the realm of Self-Directed Education. We see here how respecting children, listening to them, and learning from them can revolutionize our manner of parenting and remove the blinders imposed by the forced schooling that we nearly all experienced. I recommend it to everyone who cares about children, freedom, and the future of humanity."
—Peter Gray, research professor of psychology at Boston College, author of *Free to Learn*

Queercore: How to Punk a Revolution: An Oral History

Edited by Liam Warfield, Walter Crasshole, and Yony Leyser with an Introduction by Anna Joy Springer and Lynn Breedlove

ISBN: 978-1-62963-796-9
$20.00 208 pages

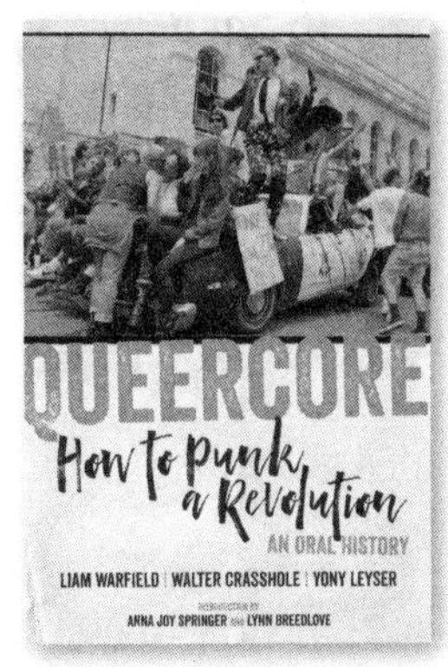

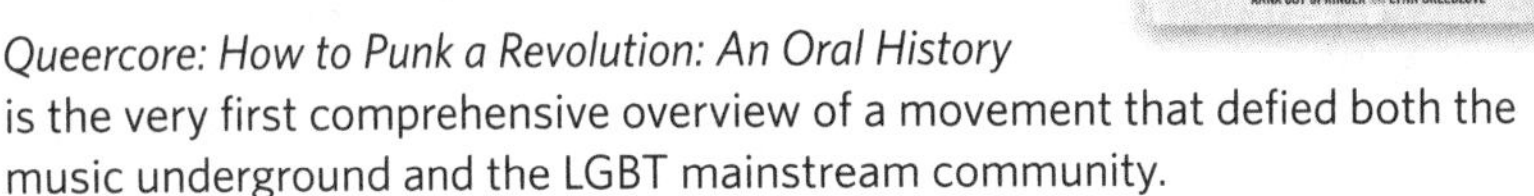
Queercore: How to Punk a Revolution: An Oral History is the very first comprehensive overview of a movement that defied both the music underground and the LGBT mainstream community.

Through exclusive interviews with protagonists like Bruce LaBruce, G.B. Jones, Jayne County, Kathleen Hanna of Bikini Kill and Le Tigre, film director and author John Waters, Lynn Breedlove of Tribe 8, Jon Ginoli of Pansy Division, and many more, alongside a treasure trove of never-before-seen photographs and reprinted zines from the time, *Queercore* traces the history of a scene originally "fabricated" in the bedrooms and coffee shops of Toronto and San Francisco by a few young, queer punks to its emergence as a relevant and real revolution. *Queercore* is a down-to-details firsthand account of the movement explored by the people that lived it—from punk's early queer elements, to the moment that Toronto kids decided they needed to create a scene that didn't exist, to Pansy Division's infiltration of the mainstream, and the emergence of riot grrrl—as well as the clothes, zines, art, film, and music that made this movement an exciting middle finger to complacent gay and straight society. *Queercore* will stand as both a testament to radically gay politics and culture and an important reference for those who wish to better understand this explosive movement.

"Finally, a book that centers on the wild, innovative, and fearless contributions queers made to punk rock, creating a punker-than-punk subculture beneath the subculture, queercore. Gossipy and inspiring, a historical document and a call to arms during a time when the entire planet could use a dose of queer, creative rage."
—Michelle Tea, author of *Valencia*

"I knew at an early age I didn't want to be part of a church, I wanted to be part of a circus. It's documents such as this book that give hope for our future. Anarchists, the queer community, the roots of punk, the Situationists, and all the other influential artistic guts eventually had to intersect. Queercore *is completely logical, relevant, and badass."*
—Justin Pearson, The Locust, Three One G

Y'all Means All: The Emerging Voices Queering Appalachia

Edited by Z. Zane McNeill

ISBN: 978-1-62963-914-7
$20.00   200 pages

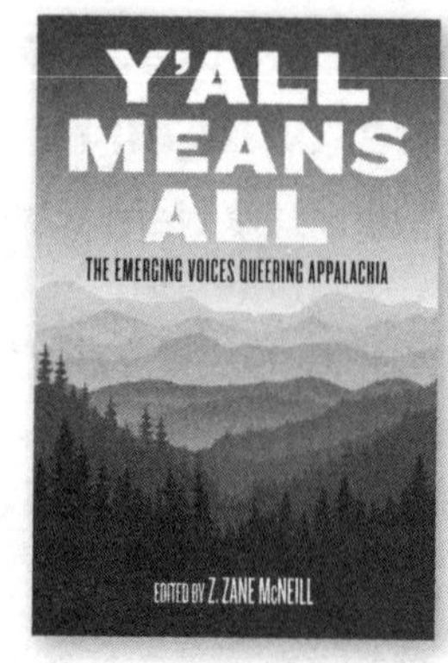

Y'all Means All is a celebration of the weird and wonderful aspects of a troubled region in all of their manifest glory! This collection is a thought-provoking hoot and a holler of "we're queer and we're here to stay, cause we're every bit a piece of the landscape as the rocks and the trees" echoing through the hills of Appalachia and into the boardrooms of every media outlet and opportunistic author seeking to define Appalachia from the outside for their own political agendas. Multidisciplinary and multi-genre, *Y'all* necessarily incorporates elements of critical theory, such as critical race theory and queer theory, while dealing with a multitude of methodologies, from quantitative analysis, to oral history and autoethnography.

This collection eschews the contemporary trend of "reactive" or "responsive" writing in the genre of Appalachian studies, and alternatively, provides examples of how modern Appalachians are defining themselves on their own terms. As such, it also serves as a toolkit for other Appalachian readers to follow suit, and similarly challenge the labels, stereotypes, and definitions often thrust upon them. While providing blunt commentary on the region's past and present, the book's soul is sustained by the resilience, ingenuity, and spirit exhibited by the authors, values which have historically characterized the Appalachian region and are continuing to define its culture to the present.

This book demonstrates above all else that Appalachia and its people are filled with a vitality and passion for their region which will slowly but surely effect long-lasting and positive changes in the region. If historically Appalachia has been treated as a "mirror" of the country, this book breaks that trend by allowing modern Appalachians to examine their own reflections and to share their insights in an honest, unfiltered manner with the world.

"These deeply personal and theoretically informed essays explore the fight for social justice and inclusivity in Appalachia through the intersections of environmental action, LGBTQA+ representational politics, anti-racism, and movements for disability justice. This Appalachia is inhabited by a queer temporality and geography, where gardening lore teaches us that seeds dance into plants in their own time, not according to a straight-edged neoliberal discipline."
—Rebecca Scott, author of *Removing Mountains: Extracting Nature and Identity in the Appalachian Coalfields*

Be Gay, Do Crime: Everyday Acts of Queer Resistance and Rebellion

Edited by Zane McNeill, Riley Clare Valentine, and Blu Buchanan with a Foreword by Cindy Barukh Milstein and an Introduction by Working Class History

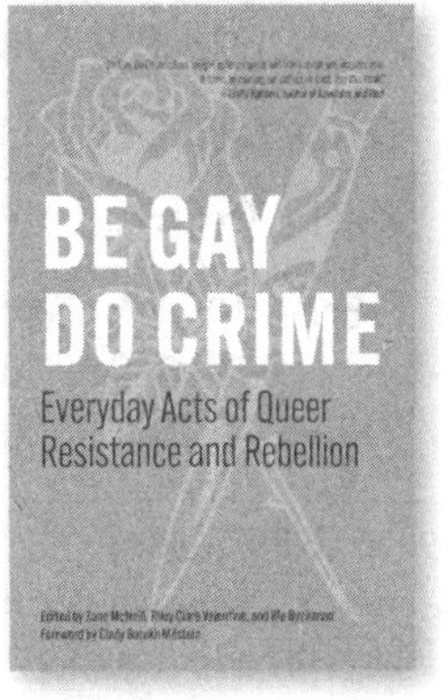

ISBN: 979-8-88744-130-6 (paperback)
979-8-88744-143-6 (hardcover)
$24.95 / $49.95 304 pages

Sometimes it pays to be gay and do crime.

As communities are boldly rising to challenge capitalism, white supremacy, and authoritarianism, *Be Gay, Do Crime: Everyday Acts of Queer Resistance and Rebellion* is your ultimate guide to LGBTQ+ resilience and rebellion. Packed with daily snapshots of radical queer history, this book celebrates the bold, the brave, and the beautifully defiant moments that have shaped the fight for justice.

Ever wonder why the Stonewall protests became an uprising or what the earliest acts of queer resistance looked like? How about the ways queer communities have organized against oppression across the globe? *Be Gay, Do Crime* dives into these stories and so many more—from fierce acts of resistance to joyful victories—bringing to life the rich, diverse history of LGBTQ+ liberation.

By situating readers within a larger pattern of struggle, these everyday acts counter the erasure of queer people from history and serve as a reminder that our struggles are part of a broader fight against systemic violence and dehumanization.

But, this isn't just a history book; it's a rallying cry. Flip to any page, soak up some inspiration, and join the legacy of resistance.

"The history of queer people is marked by resistance and resilience against significant hostility and harassment from those in power. Be Gay, Do Crime *explores the strategic use of arrests and police violence as tools to suppress individuals who bravely refused to go back into the closet. This almanac highlights incredible acts of defiance in the face of power and shows us all on whose shoulders we stand."*
—Erin Reed, transgender activist and journalist

"Day by day, the collective vigilance of queer people in the US and around the world has led us on paths toward liberation. This book of days names the names—some renowned and many forgotten—and celebrates quotidian victories, one day at a time. This daybook is a keeper!"
—Rahne Alexander, intermedia artist and writer from Baltimore

A People's Guide to Abolition and Disability Justice

Katie Tastrom

ISBN: 979-8-88744-040-8 (paperback)
979-8-88744-054-5 (hardcover)
$19.95 / $29.95 256 pages

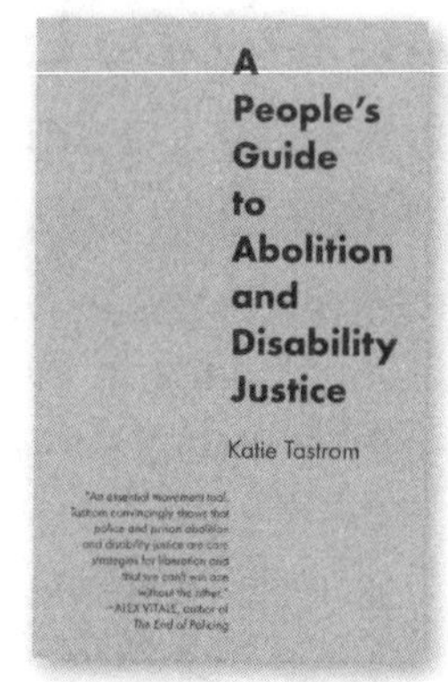

Disability justice and prison abolition are two increasingly popular theories that overlap but whose intersection has rarely been explored in depth.

A People's Guide to Abolition and Disability Justice explains the history and theories behind abolition and disability justice in a way that is easy to understand for those new to these concepts yet also gives insights that will be useful to seasoned activists. The book uses extensive research and professional and lived experience to illuminate the way the State uses disability and its power to disable to incarcerate multiply marginalized disabled people, especially those who are queer, trans, Black, or Indigenous.

Because disabled people are much more likely than nondisabled people to be locked up in prisons, jails, and other sites of incarceration, abolitionists and others critical of carceral systems must incorporate a disability justice perspective into our work. *A People's Guide to Abolition and Disability Justice* gives personal and policy examples of how and why disabled people are disproportionately caught up in the carceral net, and how we can use this information to work toward prison and police abolition more effectively. This book includes practical tools and strategies that will be useful for anyone who cares about disability justice or abolition and explains why we can't have one without the other.

"An essential movement tool. Tastrom convincingly shows that police and prison abolition and disability justice are core strategies for liberation and that we can't win one without the other."
—Alex Vitale, professor of sociology and coordinator of the Policing and Social Justice Project at Brooklyn College and the CUNY Graduate Center, and author of *City of Disorder* and *The End of Policing*

"A People's Guide to Abolition and Disability Justice *is a clear, accessible, and invaluable tool for not only dissecting the depths of disability and criminalization but also illustrating how the fights for disability justice and prison abolition are inextricably linked."*
—Victoria Law, author of *Resistance Behind Bars: The Struggles of Incarcerated Women* and *"Prisons Make Us Safer" & 20 Other Myths About Mass Incarceration*